T0144657

BASIC HEALTH PUBLICATIONS USER'S GUIDE

TO TREATING HEPATITIS NATURALLY

Learn How Supplements Can Reverse Symptoms of Hepatitis and Improve Your Health.

DOUGLAS MACKAY, N.D.

JACK CHALLEM Series Editor

Series Editor: Jack Challem
Editor: Jane E. Morrill
Typesetter: Gary A. Rosenberg
Series Cover Designer: Mike Stromberg

Basic Health Publications User's Guides are published by Basic Health Publications, Inc.

CONTENTS

INTRODUCTION

L-I-V-E: Without a doubt the first four letters of the word "liver" say it all. The liver is a major organ of digestion responsible for the assimilation and removal of toxic waste from the body. Unfortunately, liver diseases, such as hepatitis, are the fourth-leading cause of death in the United States.

Hepatitis is a generic term that combines the word "hepatic," referring to the liver, and "itis," a medical suffix meaning inflammation. Together, "hepatitis" means "an inflammatory condition of the liver." It is considered a generic term because there are several underlying factors that can cause the inflammation. Bacterial or viral infection, parasitic infection, alcohol, drugs, and toxins can all result in hepatitis. The disease can last for a week or linger for a lifetime, depending on the specific cause.

Hepatitis C, a type of viral hepatitis, is the most common cause of liver disease in Western nations. It has been estimated that 175 million people worldwide are infected with the hepatitis C virus (HCV), including approximately 3 to 4 million people in the United States. Sound bad? It gets worse. Deaths from hepatitis C are expected to triple in the next five to ten years.

Current management of hepatitis C includes drugs that have severe side effects and unsatisfactory cure rates. All practitioners and patients familiar with the relentless nature of hepatitis C can agree on one thing: Alternative and more effective therapies are needed for the treatment of hepatitis C.

Successful nutritional, herbal, and dietary approaches to hepatitis C are in use throughout the world. Unfortunately, not all available treatment strategies are universally presented to hepatitis C–positive individuals. If you are interested in learning about effective, nontoxic, complementary and alternative approaches to the management of hepatitis C, read on!

This *User's Guide to Treating Hepatitis Naturally* is a thorough guidebook that will help you to understand this confusing topic. The book focuses on hepatitis C and complementary and alternative treatments for it. Chapters 1 through 3 provide a foundation for understanding hepatitis, including its effect on the liver, various underlying causes, and its various means of transmission.

The second half of this user's guide is dedicated to complementary and alternative treatments for hepatitis C. Chapter 4 explores diet and lifestyle issues that profoundly impact hepatitis patients, yet are seldom discussed by doctors. Chapter 5 focuses on vitamins, minerals, and other nutrients used to manage this disease. Chapter 6 is dedicated to herbal medicines shown to be effective for it. The final chapter provides a summary of the information presented in the book.

The *User's Guide to Treating Hepatitis Naturally* presents a balanced approach to hepatitis C with an emphasis on science-based nutritional and herbal treatments. It is not meant to replace a doctor's medical advice, but rather to educate readers about the many valuable—and often ignored—treatments available to hepatitis patients.

Beating hepatitis C is tough. Conventional and alternative doctors struggle to provide the best treatments for their patients. As you will discover, the best management of hepatitis C includes a combination of the therapies offered by both conventional and alternative disciplines.

CHAPTER 1

FACTS ABOUT
THE LIVER

For most people the liver is a complex and mysterious organ. It has thousands of intricate biochemical functions that even scientists do not fully understand. To fully appreciate the widespread effects of hepatitis on health and well-being, it's necessary to explore basic information about the liver. This chapter covers the basic functions of the liver while providing a foundation to better understand the impact of hepatitis on overall health.

The Importance of the Liver

The liver is one of the largest and most important organs in the body. More than 5,000 of the liver's functions have been identified, and scientists are still discovering new ones. The liver, like the heart and lungs, is essential for survival.

Obviously, all of the body's organs are important. There are, however, some organs that can be considered essential. Ask ten random people off the street what their most vital organs are, and most would respond: brain, heart, and lungs.

The relative importance of the liver is illustrated by a few simple facts. The liver first appears at three-weeks' gestation and begins to contribute to fetal survival at six-weeks' gestation. Making red blood cells is one the liver's first big jobs, one that it does until the bone marrow takes over this critical task.

The liver receives 20 percent of all the blood pumped by the heart. Two separate sources supply blood to the liver. One brings oxygen-rich blood from the lungs to nourish liver cells. The other brings blood from the stomach and intestines loaded with the products of digestion. The liver is responsible for absorbing, sorting, and processing all nutrients. It is also responsible for eliminating all toxins and waste. This is a huge amount of work for one organ.

A final fact that demonstrates the liver's relative importance is how the body has evolved to protect this vital organ. Have you ever noticed that all the critical organs are encased in bone for protection? Just as the brain is surrounded by the skull, the liver is guarded on all sides by the ribcage.

The Location of the Liver

Sternum
The elongated, flattened bone that forms the middle portion of the chest cavity, situated between the lungs.

The liver is located in the upper-right abdomen and is encased by the ribcage. The lower border of the liver starts at the sternum and runs along the lower-right rib, out to the side. From its lower edge, the liver spans upward 6–12 centimeters.

The liver responds to disease by either increasing or decreasing in size. During a physical exam doctors try to determine the liver's size by digging their fingers under the right ribcage. This is a fairly uncomfortable way to locate the lower border of the liver; hopefully, it won't be found.

The lower border of the liver should not be felt if you have a healthy liver. When the liver is challenged by disease, it enlarges beyond its protective cavity. This pushes the liver's lower edge within reach of a doctor's fingers. A surface that should be firm and smooth can sometimes become flabby, nodular, or irregular.

The Function of the Liver

The liver is a solid organ that weighs 1,200–1,500

hardworking grams. It is essentially the most efficient factory ever built. The liver is divided into four compartments, or "lobes," which are further divided into 100,000 smaller compartments, or "lobules."

Imagine a factory with 100,000 departments that creates 500,000 different parts, which are used to complete more than 5,000 different tasks. In addition, this factory has storage and shipping departments and weighs only 1,500 grams. This factory is the liver.

There are millions of cell membranes within the liver. These membranes direct the movement, filtration, and storage of thousands of tiny compounds. Oxidative damage to cell membranes within the liver plays a major role in damaging these compounds and ultimately in developing chronic liver disease.

Liver cells are known as "hepatocytes" and account for 60 percent of total liver mass. They are responsible for molecular synthesis, carbohydrate metabolism, fat metabolism, blood detoxification, and the formation of bile.

Nutrient-rich blood from the digestive system does not come into direct contact with the hepatocytes. A one-cell-thick barrier exists between the blood and the hepatocyte. This area is known as the "spaces of Disse," and it prefilters the blood before it arrives at the hepatocyte.

Phagocytosis
Ingestion and digestion of bacteria, viruses, or toxins by cells designed to consume and destroy invading substances.

Another very important type of cell, the Kupffer's cell, is exposed to the blood before the liver cells are. Kupffer's cells are responsible for the phagocytic activity of blood-borne products delivered to the liver. Normally small and inconspicuous, Kupffer's cells undergo enlargement in response to a toxin or an invading organism.

As you can see, the liver takes detoxification very seriously. Liver cells provide the backbone of detoxification. However, the blood must overcome two protective layers before it even contacts the liver cells.

Throughout the liver is a sophisticated plumbing system that transports blood, lymph, and bile separately. The bile system transports and actively modifies about one liter of bile daily. Lymphatic channels gather and drain excess fluid that has collected in the spaces of Disse. Running parallel to these two systems, the vascular system filters more than a liter of blood per minute.

Bile
A bitter, yellow-green secretion of the liver that is stored in the gallbladder and used to emulsify fat in the diet.

If the liver doesn't amaze you by the sheer complexity of its organization, just wait! The number of different jobs the liver is responsible for is downright baffling.

The liver synthesizes and metabolizes essential compounds for the body. Nutrients and compounds manufactured by the liver are stored and released based on the body's needs. This job alone requires an advanced communication system that runs among the liver and other organs. In addition, the liver manages to save enough time and space to clear drugs and toxins from the system. To extract dietary nutrients, the liver must also remove potentially harmful compounds and bacteria that occur naturally. In addition, the liver must eliminate environmental toxins absorbed from the air, food, and water.

Metabolism
Chemical processes resulting in growth, generation of energy, elimination of waste, and other bodily functions, as they relate to the distribution of nutrients in the blood.

A laundry list of the liver's primary functions includes the following; it:

- Stores vitamins, minerals, and sugars.
- Filters the blood, removing harmful substances.
- Creates bile, which is essential for fat digestion.
- Metabolizes proteins, fats, and carbo-hydrates.
- Absorbs and stores the fat-soluble vitamins (A, D, E, and K).
- Synthesizes valuable immune-system compounds.
- Processes and eliminates excess hormones and toxins.
- Stores extra blood.

The liver accomplishes these tasks with the help of thousands of enzymes. Liver enzymes are arranged in assembly lines that create or break down substances based on the body's ever-chang-ing needs. The liver stays informed of the body's needs by constant input from various nerves, sig-naling molecules, and hormones.

Enzyme
A protein that facilitates chemical reactions in organic matter.

The Liver and Detoxification

Detoxification, the rendering of a poisonous sub-stance into something harmless, is arguably one of the most important functions of the liver. We are exposed to many toxic compounds, both nat-ural and unnatural, on a daily basis. These com-pounds must be processed and disposed of. The liver deactivates and removes all substances that should not be absorbed.

A normal diet contains small amounts of natu-ral toxins. We never even know that we ingest these poisons because the liver takes care of metabolizing and excreting them. If these toxins were allowed to accumulate, they would cause metabolic mayhem.

The same holds true for countless toxins resulting from the industrial revolution and our modern lifestyles. Unfortunately, the human body is not equipped to handle large amounts of highly toxic synthetic compounds. The result has been a series of new diseases such as multiple-chemical-sensitivity syndrome and sick-building syndrome.

Multiple-Chemical-Sensitivity Syndrome
Unusual, and sometimes intense, adverse physical reactions to common synthetic chemicals, such as cleaning solutions and carpets.

Sick-Building Syndrome
An illness that a building's occupants may fall victim to that is caused by the synthetic chemicals, glues, and paints used during its construction.

The liver detoxifies harmful compounds by creating assembly lines of enzymes. These enzymes make chemical changes to toxic compounds, rendering them harmless. Researchers have discovered that enzymatic detoxification occurs in two phases.

Phase One and Phase Two Detoxification Pathways

The phases of liver detoxification have been not-so-creatively named "phase one" and "phase two." In phase one, a series of enzymatic reactions render the starting toxic compound more soluble in water, thus aiding its removal from the body. In phase two, a series of enzymatic reactions attach, or "conjugate," the starting toxic compound to a second compound that deactivates or nullifies the toxin.

For biochemistry enthusiasts, phase one reactions use a family of enzymes known as the "cytochrome P-450" enzymes. This is a complex system that is under genetic control. Cytochrome

P-450 enzymes are also highly sensitive to stimulation or inhibition by many factors. For example, stimulation of phase one enzymes allows the liver to metabolize a larger amount of toxic compounds more efficiently. This explains why alcoholics have such a high tolerance to sedatives and other agents metabolized along the same pathway. Inhibition of the cytochrome P-450 enzymes reduces the liver's ability to metabolize harmful compounds. This can occur as a result of external factors such as drugs, diet, smoking, and caffeine. Thus, the liver's ability to metabolize toxins varies widely among healthy individuals.

Phase two deactivates the toxin by attaching a second compound to the parent, or original, compound. This is the unifying principle among phase two reactions. It is analogous to attaching a muzzle to a vicious dog to make it less likely to bite a neighbor.

Glutathione

Glutathione is the universal detoxifier. All the cells in the body contain glutathione as part of the phase two detoxification system. The liver, as the master organ of detoxification, is the body's largest reservoir of glutathione.

Glutathione levels are considered a sensitive indicator of cell function and viability. If these levels are depleted, progressive loss of cell function results and can ultimately lead to cell death. Chronic disease is known to deplete glutathione levels.

Glutathione plays a large role in detoxifying prescription drugs by binding to potentially hazardous intermediate compounds. If this mechanism is saturated by too much medication, as in the case of drug overload, then the resulting free intermediate compounds bind to the liver cells. The resulting liver damage may not show up for a couple of days, but when it does, acute liver failure occurs.

Hepatitis delivers a double whammy in relation to glutathione. Suarez et al. showed that viral hepatitis depletes liver glutathione levels. Since the glutathione reservoir for the whole body is found in the liver, the threat to cell function and viability is not limited to that organ.

Glutathione depletion can account for the multisystem nature of hepatitis symptoms, such as nausea, vomiting, and fatigue. In addition, studies have shown that glutathione depletion is linked to the progression of hepatitis to cirrhosis and liver failure. The good news is: Safe and effective nutritional supplements have been shown to raise glutathione levels.

Phase One and Phase Two at Work

An example of this highly efficient detoxification mechanism is shown by the ongoing neutralization of ammonium ions created within the body. Poisonous ammonium ions are created as byproducts of the transformation of protein into energy. Ammonium is sent to the liver where phase one and phase two enzyme systems convert this potential poison into the innocuous compound "urea," which is passed to the urine for excretion.

Ammonium Ion
An ion formed, in this context, as a waste product of protein metabolism.

The timing of phase one and phase two reactions can be delicate. In some instances the result of phase one reactions is an intermediate molecule that is more toxic than its parent compound. A good example of this is the metabolism of alcohol.

Hypotension
An abnormal condition in which the blood pressure is too low for normal perfusion and oxygenation of the tissues.

The metabolism of alcohol takes place in the liver. Phase one enzymes metabolize alcohol into "acetaldehyde." Acetaldehyde is toxic to humans and causes flushing, headache, nausea, vomiting, sweating, and hypotension. Luck-

ily, in phase two reactions, the liver quickly transforms acetaldehyde into acetate, which is harmless and easy to eliminate.

A genetic variation found in 50 percent of
Asians deactivates the enzyme that is responsible for transforming acetaldehyde to acetate.
This causes some Asians to experience flushing
and other unpleasant effects when consuming
small amounts of alcohol. It is also an example of
genetic individuality.

The phase one and phase two enzymes in each
genetic background are unique. One compound
may be poisonous to one particular genetic
makeup and benign to another. It's common for
pharmaceutical drugs to have adverse effects in a
particular subset of the population, indicating
that certain people do not have the correct
enzymes to metabolize a drug.

Understanding phase one and phase two
metabolism has led to the development of
drugs that can manipulate individual enzymes
to achieve a desired outcome. Disulfiram (Antabuse), a drug prescribed for alcohol abuse or
alcoholism, blocks the phase two enzymes responsible for transforming acetaldehyde into acetate.
Similar to what is seen in some Asians, Antabuse
causes a violent reaction with just a small amount
of alcohol.

The biochemistry that underlies liver detoxification is complex. It is also dynamic, able to
respond to ever-changing challenges. As we age
and environmental consequences become more
inevitable, our livers will be forced to adapt.

The Liver Faces Great Challenges

Modern lifestyles have introduced many new
challenges for the liver. Environmental toxins,
food chemicals, the use of alcohol, caffeine, and
nicotine, and high levels of stress produce toxins
that the liver must handle. Even in a pristine envi-

ronment, the job of extracting nutrients, while breaking down and eliminating toxins, is complex. Add to this a modern lifestyle, and it's no surprise that liver disease is rising at epidemic proportions.

Processed foods alone contain preservatives, coloring agents, pesticides, herbicides, and synthetic sweeteners and oils. The average American ingests thousands of synthetic chemicals every year. These compounds are completely new and different from the natural compounds that the liver has evolved metabolizing.

Chemical companies are responsible for creating thousands of new chemicals per year. Many of these chemicals are designed as additives for food and prescription medicines. Other compounds are developed for industrial use and released into the air and water as pollution.

Federal Superfund Site

Our nation's worst toxic-waste sites eligible for long-term remediation, which seeks to permanently and significantly reduce the volume, toxicity, or mobility of the toxic contaminants in the waste.

Toxins known to pass through the liver include herbicides and pesticides, including DDT, dioxins, PCBs, and PCPs. More than 4 *billion* pounds of toxic chemicals are released by industry into the environment of the United States each year, including 72 million pounds of recognized cancer-causing agents. About 11 million people in the United States, including 3 to 4 million children, live within one mile of a federal superfund site and are exposed to potential public-health risks.

It has become necessary for all humans to detoxify regularly to maintain health and vitality. Cleansing and detoxification are also important to clear symptoms and treat chronic disease. In viral hepatitis it is particularly important to eliminate excess toxins by eliminating such habits as consuming alcohol, caffeine, and nicotine.

In addition to stopping behaviors that expose the body to excess toxins, facilitating the removal of environmental toxins from the liver is imperative. Chapters 5 and 6 cover nutrients and herbs used to clear this toxic buildup from the liver.

Toxins and Viral Hepatitis

The connection between increases in toxicity and increases in disease seems obvious. However, the connection between increased toxicity and increased incidence of hepatitis is often ignored.

Chris Metro, a naturopathic doctor and acupuncturist from Oregon, speculates that susceptibility to viral hepatitis has dramatically increased as a result of excess environmental and dietary toxins. Dr. Metro points out that hepatitis viruses are not new, yet deaths from hepatitis C alone are expected to triple in the next five to ten years. Why is hepatitis on the rise? If the liver were not overloaded with toxic buildup, it might be able to eliminate the virus more successfully.

Currently, one quarter of the people who contract a hepatitis virus clear it without long-term effects. Could it be that in the past this number was greater?

It has been suggested that the hepatitis C virus (HCV) is a latent virus that has lived inside of humans since early existence. Unhealthy lifestyles and environmental toxins may have triggered its reappearance. Toxins are known to deteriorate the immune system, which is thought to allow the virus to propagate.

Drug companies are feverishly pursuing medicines that will kill viral hepatitis. This is important. However, it is equally important to focus on the health of the liver where the virus is trying to make its home. Improving liver function and decreasing the load of built-up toxins reduces the probability that the virus can survive in the liver.

The Liver and the Emotions

The liver transforms and removes excess hormones from the blood. The ancient healing systems of both India and China established a correlation between the liver and emotional well-being more than 2,000 years ago. This was long before people understood the liver's anatomy, physiology, or biochemistry.

The liver is perhaps the most congested of all the organs in the modern person. Too many chemicals, stimulants, intoxicants, and synthetic foods and too much fat disrupt the liver's intricate processing, including the metabolism of hormones. This can affect routine tasks such as the conjugation and excretion of hormones.

The first sign of liver disharmony is emotional difficulty related to anger. It is common for hepatitis patients to experience mood swings, impatience, frustration, aggression, depression, impulsiveness, or other emotional challenges. A healthy liver facilitates a calm, centered state of being.

It's not uncommon for a doctor to prescribe antidepressants or antianxiety medications for hepatitis patients. Although these medicines may mask the emotional symptoms, they give the liver more drugs to detoxify. This further congests the organ, leading to greater liver disharmony and more emotional difficulty.

CHAPTER 2

WHEN INFLAMMATION STRIKES THE LIVER

Inflammation is a basic physiologic response to injury. Researchers are finding that it is also an underlying component of most chronic diseases. Chronic hepatitis is no different. This chapter explores how viruses, chemicals, alcohol, and other causes of hepatitis all result in inflammation of the liver, which leads to chronic liver disease.

The Liver and Inflammation—Hepatitis

The liver detoxifies toxins, viruses, bacteria, and other substances in a similar fashion. Liver-cell size, number, and activity increase, resulting in generalized inflammation. Part of this response includes mobilizing cells to capture the offender. The Kupffer's cells gobble up toxic compounds and package them into membranes for neutralization. Enzymes neutralize packaged toxins and prepare them for removal.

When toxic exposure increases, the liver recruits more enzymes in an effort to keep up with the load. If liver enzymes are being recruited to handle large amounts of toxic material, other metabolic jobs are being neglected. One of the first jobs interrupted is the production of bile. Disruption of this process causes bilirubin, the yellow pigment in bile, to build up. The yellow pigment spills into the tissue and causes yellowing of the skin, eyes, and

Jaundice
Yellowing of the skin, eyes, and mucous membranes, a condition caused by disturbances in the functioning of liver cells.

mucous membranes, creating a condition known as jaundice.

If the liver cannot keep up with the volume of toxins it is being exposed to, it recruits more immune and inflammatory cells. Inflammatory cells present a double-edged sword to the liver. On one hand, inflammatory cells are capable of capturing, killing, and neutralizing the invader. On the other hand, inflammation is a process that results in copious free-radical production. Without adequate antioxidant protection, significant cellular damage can occur.

Inflammation is an example of a nonspecific immune response to infection or injury. For example, a sprained ankle results in pain, swelling, and a reduced range of motion. This inflammatory process removes damaged tissue, allows for rest, and brings in cellular building blocks for repair.

Nonspecific Immune Response
Initial immune reaction to injury and disease that is not disease-specific and is characterized by fever, inflammation, and increased blood supply.

Sounds good, right? However, in conditions such as arthritis, inflammation can become long term, and long-term inflammation in the joint space generates an excess of free radicals. This, in turn, causes damage, erosion, fibrosis, and loss of function to the joint.

The liver responds in a similar way. A short-term challenge may temporarily cause pain and enlargement of the liver, as well as elevated liver-function tests. Damage from this stage of injury is reversible. If the problem persists, however, fatty and fibrous tissue begins to replace healthy cells, resulting in a loss of function. This is known as cirrhosis of the liver.

Cirrhosis
Degenerative disease of the liver where liver tissue is replaced by fibrous scarring and the liver hardens and loses function.

Causes of Hepatitis

Hepatitis can be caused by a variety of different instigators: toxins, viruses, bacteria, alcohol, drugs, and more. Let's explore some of them.

Alcoholic Hepatitis

It is common knowledge that alcohol damages the liver. Alcohol is a solvent, and like any other solvent, it must be metabolized and eliminated. Alcohol in excess over a period of time leads to the development of fatty deposits within the liver.

Solvent
Any liquid in which another substance can be dissolved.

This stage of alcoholic hepatitis is known as "fatty liver" and is reversible. Strict abstinence from alcohol at this stage can lead to full recovery.

When individuals with fatty liver choose not to quit drinking, the fat in the liver cells begins to cause inflammation. This is known as alcoholic hepatitis. If drinking continues, this condition progresses to scarring and hardening of the liver, known as cirrhosis. Unlike other forms of hepatitis, the treatment for alcoholic hepatitis is straightforward. If the patient stops drinking before permanent damage sets in, the liver will regenerate.

In the United States one of the main causes of liver cirrhosis is excess alcohol consumption over many years. For most people this is not a concern because they are in control of their alcohol consumption. Unfortunately, our modern lifestyles have introduced other substances equally as challenging for the liver.

Drug-Induced/Toxic Hepatitis

Long-term use of the mild painkiller acetaminophen (Tylenol) can cause chronic liver disease and even death. Acute overdose of this over-the-counter "wonder drug" has become a prominent cause of fulminant liver failure. And they say that herbs and vitamins are dangerous!

**Fulminant
Liver Failure**
*A frequently fatal
form of hepatitis in
which there is rapid
deterioration in the
condition of the
patient.*

Drugs are an important cause of hepatitis. The mechanisms by which drugs cause hepatitis are variable and in most instances poorly understood. Drugs are synthetic chemicals that the liver needs to remove from the body. Drug-induced hepatitis occurs when the combined load of prescribed drugs and other toxins exceeds the liver's detoxification capacity. This situation can easily occur, considering that many people are on multiple drugs and live in a toxic environment.

Scientists have discovered that certain drugs are directly toxic to the liver. These drugs are essentially poisonous. For these drugs, liver injury is generally predictable and dose-related.

Drugs Known to Cause Hepatitis

- Methyldopa
- Isoniazid
- Nitrofurantoin
- Acetaminophen

**Idiosyncratic
Drug Reaction**
*An unusual response
to a drug that manifests as an accelerated,
toxic, or inappropriate
response to its usual
therapeutic dose.*

Other drugs cause an idiosyncratic reaction. In other words, we have no idea why a particular drug is damaging to some individuals and not to others. Taking multiple powerful medications can become a form of Russian roulette.

Idiosyncratic drug reactions are beyond the scope of this user's guide. However, they bring up two important considerations: total load and genetic variability.

Total Load and Genetic Variability

When doctors look for the cause of hepatitis, they are usually in search of one causative agent.

Is it a drug, a virus, or alcohol? Consider someone whose liver is metabolizing all three.

Cytochrome P-450 enzymes are inhibited by external factors such as alcohol, caffeine, and cigarettes. Take a person with all three of these habits, and give them three prescriptions. I say, the total is greater than the sum of the parts, not "idiosyncratic drug reaction."

As I mentioned earlier, the over-the-counter painkiller acetaminophen can cause acute hepatitis. A dose much lower than normal has the same effect in alcoholics. In this example, the total load includes acetaminophen and alcohol, which reduces the cytochrome P-450 activity and depletes glutathione levels.

Genetic variability is the second factor that reduces predictability in liver disease. The types and subtypes of cytochrome P-450 in each of us are unique, giving each of us different detoxification capabilities.

Inborn metabolism errors are clear examples of how minor differences in genes can have major effects. One or two gene differences can result in an inability to metabolize essential amino acids. Phenylketonuria (PKU) is such a condition, one that can result in severe mental retardation. In this case, a minor difference in liver metabolism can cause an essential nutrient to become a poison.

Nonalcoholic Steatohepatitis (NASH)

NASH, or nonalcoholic fatty liver, is a progressive liver disease that is becoming increasingly recognized worldwide. Patients present liver findings that are consistent with viral or alcoholic liver disease in the absence of a viral infection or a history of alcohol overuse.

What concerns doctors about NASH is that it is a progressive disease. Just like other forms of hepatitis, the disease is initiated by the presence of fat in the liver cells (steatosis). There would be no cause for alarm if NASH stopped there. Unfortunately, following steatosis, there is inflammation and fibrosis. If this isn't stopped, it can progress to cirrhosis and liver failure. The alarming fact is that 50 percent of those patients with NASH that started as simple steatosis, progress to liver fibrosis; 15 to 30 percent of them progress to cirrhosis; and 3 percent experience liver failure.

You may be asking yourself, in the absence of alcohol or a virus, what's going on here? It appears that NASH is merely another aspect of "metabolic syndrome," or Syndrome X. The cornerstone of Syndrome X is obesity and insulin resistance. In a nutshell, obesity and insulin resistance lead to an alteration in fat metabolism and an increase in oxidative stress. This creates inflammation and fibrosis, which generates more free radicals. Here we find the mechanism underlying all chronic liver disease playing itself out.

Hepatitis A (HAV)

Hepatitis A, a liver disease caused by HAV, is highly contagious and most commonly found in areas of overcrowding and poor sanitation. The virus is transmitted via infected feces into the food or water supply. In developed countries, hepatitis A can be acquired from contaminated raw seafood or within institutions and day-care facilities.

HAV attacks the liver fast and hard, causing acute hepatitis. Unlike other types of viral hepatitis, hepatitis A usually resolves in four to six weeks and does not cause long-lasting liver disease.

Some individuals exposed to HAV will have minor or unnoticed symptoms. The immune system kills and removes the virus before it does any harm. Less fortunate individuals will experience symptoms that are indistinguishable from other types of hepatitis and last for several weeks.

Hepatitis B (HBV)

Hepatitis B is a liver disease caused by HBV. It can be a serious form of viral hepatitis. The virus is transmitted via contaminated blood, feces, or other human secretions. Professionals such as nurses, doctors, laboratory workers, and dentists who come into contact with blood and tissue are at risk for contracting the disease. However, medical professionals are not the only ones at risk for hepatitis B. High-risk behaviors such as unprotected sex and intravenous (IV) drug use also pose a significant risk for contracting hepatitis B.

High-Risk Behaviors for Contracting Hepatitis B

- IV drug use
- Unprotected sex

Significant progress has been made in controlling the spread of HBV. Its transmission has been reduced by screening donated blood, sterilizing medical equipment, and providing safe-sex education programs. Other programs have aimed to reduce IV drug use and educate users on ways to reduce their risk of getting hepatitis.

A vaccination for hepatitis B is available for healthcare workers and other individuals at high risk for contracting the virus. Hepatitis C patients should also be vaccinated for hepatitis B. Infection with both viruses is *definitely* something to avoid.

Hepatitis B can be serious and potentially fatal. However, less than 10 percent of infected adults fail to clear the virus from the body.

Hepatitis C Virus (HCV)

Hepatitis C is a liver disease caused by HCV. It is spread when blood or body fluids from an infected person enter the body of a person who is not infected. This could occur through sharing needles, needlesticks, blood transfusion, kidney dialysis, or during the birth process.

Approximately 75 percent of hepatitis C patients struggle with the virus for a lifetime. All types of viral hepatitis pose a risk to health; however, the next chapter explores why hepatitis C presents a unique challenge.

Hepatitis D Virus (HDV)

Hepatitis D is a liver disease caused by HDV, a defective virus found in the blood that requires HBV to exist. Hepatitis D is a serious and potentially life-threatening disease. Chronic HDV infection may result in the need for a liver transplant.

HDV is transmitted by contact with bodily fluids, such as through IV drug usage and unprotected sex or through needlesticks during various health procedures. Hepatitis D is often found as a coinfection or superinfection with hepatitis B. Routine statistical data on the prevalence of HDV infection is not yet available.

Hepatitis E Virus (HEV)

Hepatitis E is a liver disease caused by HEV, which is transmitted in much the same way as HAV. Hepatitis E, however, does not occur often in the United States. Although hepatitis E is uncommon in the United States, it can be a serious concern for pregnant women in their third trimester of pregnancy. Fetal loss is common. Fatality rates as high as 15 to 25 percent have been reported among pregnant women who contract HEV. Hepatitis E is typically found in people between the ages of fifteen and forty.

HEV is transmitted by contact with contaminated food, water, or feces. Contaminated drinking water is the most common cause in developing countries. To prevent infection, always wash your hands after using the bathroom or changing a diaper, and before preparing food. Also, avoid water and raw foods of unknown cleanliness.

Hepatitis E has only an acute phase and can be identified only by serologic testing.

Symptoms of Hepatitis

The word "hepatitis" is accurate regardless of the cause. Because the liver's biochemical response to various invaders is the same, symptoms of hepatitis from any cause are generally very similar.

Acute Phase

Acute hepatitis can cause severe and debilitating symptoms. These symptoms, however, last for only a relatively short period of time, when compared to chronic hepatitis. Acute hepatitis can result from a variety of causes, such as viruses, drugs, or parasites.

Acute
Starting abruptly with high intensity and subsiding after a short period of time.

When hit with acute hepatitis, the experience includes a sudden onset of fatigue, loss of appetite, nausea, and vomiting. Distaste for cigarettes and second-hand smoke usually accompanies this stage. It's interesting how the body knows when enough is enough.

Rashes and joint pain can follow the initial symptoms. After three to ten days, dark urine appears, which is a sign that the liver is struggling to keep up with its routine metabolic work. Last, the skin, eyes, and mucous membranes take on a characteristic yellow appearance, signaling jaundice.

Jaundice peaks within one to two weeks of the initial onset of symptoms, and it fades over a two-to-four-week recovery period. All forms of viral hepatitis, including hepatitis A, B, C, D, and E, have an acute stage. The big difference is that hepatitis A and B are usually cleared from the body after the acute phase, and no chronic phase has yet been identified for hepatitis E.

Chronic Phase

In between acute hepatitis and cirrhosis is chronic hepatitis. The textbook definition of chronic hepatitis is hepatitis that lasts for more than six months. The virus, unfortunately, never read the textbook. Chronic hepatitis affects people in a myriad of different ways. There are, however, two main groupings for chronic hepatitis.

General Symptoms of Hepatitis

- Loss of appetite
- Fever
- Nausea
- Vomiting
- Fatigue
- Flu-like symptoms
- Enlarged liver
- Jaundice
- Dark urine
- Elevated liver enzymes

Chronic *persistent* hepatitis usually follows acute hepatitis. Elevated liver enzymes persist in the absence of other symptoms. Orthodox medicine has determined this to be a benign condition and suggests that no treatment is necessary.

This is absurd! During chronic persistent hepatitis, the liver is working hard to completely eliminate the virus and toxins. Anytime the liver is working overtime, it is our job to provide support through proper nutrition and gentle detoxification.

Chronic *active* hepatitis is an aggressive type of hepatitis that can result in liver failure and cirrhosis. HCV is a major cause of chronic active hepatitis. Other causes include medication, other diseases, and the ever-present "unknown cause." Currently, thousands of people suffer from hepatitis with no known causative agent, known as NASH.

The symptoms of chronic active hepatitis vary. Most people experience nonspecific discomfort, uneasiness, tiredness, weakness, and loss of appetite. A subset of people will also experience low-grade fever, abdominal discomfort, nausea, vomiting, and muscle pain.

These symptoms may progress to jaundice, light stool, and a tender and enlarged liver. This stage can result in abdominal bloating, enlarged spleen, and spider veins (found above the waist, usually on the chest, upper back, shoulders, upper arms, face, and neck).

Spider Veins

A group of veins that can be seen at the surface of the skin and have a wheel-and-spoke shape that resembles a spider.

Over time the hepatitis often results in multisystem or immune symptoms. These can affect any body system and include acne, joint pain, menstrual irregularities, thyroid dysfunction, kidney problems, and more. Multisystem involvement has been classified as an "autoimmune" component of hepatitis. Translated, this means that we have no idea what's happening. The body, in a sense, has begun to work against itself.

Autoimmune

Pertaining to the development of an immune response against one's own tissues.

Hepatitis C has an insidious nature. The initial infection may be mistaken for symptoms of a common cold or flu. The patient may not realize that something is wrong until a different bodily system is affected. The multitude of ways in which hepatitis C can affect us is baffling to doctors and often results in a misdiagnosis.

Hepatitis C and Chronic Active Hepatitis

The inflammatory process in the liver, if left unchecked, can have a devastating outcome. Hepatitis C is the most common cause of liver failure and liver cancer in the West. Without the liver to clear toxins from the body, we have no chance for survival.

Liver-Function Tests

Evaluation of the functions of the liver, including key enzymes that are active in the liver. Elevation of these enzymes indicates disease.

HCV is slow to proliferate and takes a long time to cause serious disease. The infection is more often debilitating than fatal, symptoms take a long time to progress, and treatment should be started long before the damage becomes irreversible.

The health and wellness of those who get hepatitis play a major role in the outcome of the disease. Everyone with hepatitis can choose to work with variables such as diet and lifestyle in combination with herbal and nutritional therapies. These variables can direct the disease process profoundly.

Orthodox doctors are big on extensive lab testing and biopsies for diagnosis and monitoring. Drug-treatment options are less than satisfactory. There is a giant gap between when complementary and alternative treatments can help to manage this condition and when drugs become necessary. After reading this book, you should feel empowered to make the choice to support the body as it struggles to defeat the hepatitis virus. Diet, lifestyle, herbal, and nutritional therapies provide a safe and effective way protect the liver from damage.

CHAPTER 3

HEPATITIS C—
THE QUIET EPIDEMIC

Since all types of hepatitis are potentially dangerous, why is there so much concern about hepatitis C? This chapter discusses the various characteristics of the hepatitis C virus (HCV) that separate hepatitis C from other forms of the condition, including how to prevent it, how it's transmitted, and traditional and more natural means of managing it.

Hepatitis C—The Initial Response

In the 1970s Japanese doctors were puzzled about the cause of abnormally high rates of liver disease in Japan. At this time only the hepatitis A virus (HAV) and the hepatitis B virus (HBV) were known to cause inflammation in the liver. The clinical picture of this chronic liver disease was unlike any encountered before.

Doctors in other parts of the world soon began to see the same baffling clinical picture that the Japanese doctors had seen. The first pattern identified was the clustering of this new liver disease among hemophiliacs. The disease was originally named "non-A non-B hepatitis."

Patients with symptoms of hepatitis who were not diagnosed as having hepatitis A or hepatitis B were diagnosed with having non-A non-B. In 1989 HCV was first identified. This prompted the screening of blood banks and the realization that thousands of people had contracted the virus from donated blood.

At first hepatitis C was not considered a serious disease. Doctors' experience with hepatitis A and its intense but short-lived symptoms did not make them suspicious of the potential for the chronic and debilitating effects of hepatitis C. Hepatitis B could be chronic and severe, but less than 10 percent of those infected did not fully recover.

Many doctors disregarded the serious nature of hepatitis C and felt that only the weak and immune-compromised were at risk of long-term complications. They were also unaware of the ease with which HCV was transmitted. In addition, doctors didn't realize that HCV might be inactive in a person for ten to thirty years before showing any symptoms. These factors led to the quiet global propagation of hepatitis C.

As early as 1940, the first major propagation of HCV began through blood transfusions. Thirty years later, when this first group of patients began exhibiting symptoms, doctors began for the first time to see the magnitude of what they were dealing with. In about 1990 it became clear that hepatitis C was a serious and dangerous epidemic.

HCV—A Tenacious Little Bugger

HCV is a basic living organism with the sole purpose of propagating itself. It lives primarily in liver cells. HCV itself is remarkably tiny, allowing it to escape undetected for many years. It travels through the blood in very small amounts. Most of it resides safely within the cells. This makes blood tests for hepatitis C expensive and extremely difficult to perform.

Even though only small amounts reside in the blood, there are three characteristics that explain its success in moving from one host to the next. HCV is virulent, highly infectious, and resilient. To a microbiologist, these words have a very specific meaning. The *virulence* of a virus means that exposure to even a small amount of it can cause a significant disease. A *highly infectious* virus means that it passes easily from a carrier to a new host. And, *resilience* refers to how hard the virus is to kill.

How One Tiny Virus Does So Much Damage

HCV damages cells by invading them and destroying structure and function. The virus also stimulates an immune response (inflammation) that further destroys surrounding cells.

The two ways in which HCV destroys liver function are important in deciding what treatments will be effective. When the virus destroys cells directly, it is known as a *cytopathic* virus. Therapy is aimed at killing the virus itself.

In comparison, an *immunopathic* virus damages tissue as a result of the immune system trying to attack the virus. Immunopathic viruses are more difficult to treat. In addition to killing the virus, suppressing the immune response in an effort to reduce damage becomes necessary.

Treatment for an immunopathic virus can be dicey. On one hand, the immune system is needed to eradicate the virus. On the other, the immune system is being suppressed to minimize damage.

HCV is considered to be both an immunopathic and a cytopathic virus. Liver biopsies reveal both direct viral damage and signs of damage

Nonliver Symptoms Associated with Hepatitis

- Joint pains
- Night sweats
- Insomnia
- Blood sugar disorders
- Symptoms of irritable bowel syndrome
- Dizziness
- Spider veins
- Reduced libido
- PMS
- Numbness of extremities

resulting from inflammation. Immunopathic viruses are also responsible for a range of associated symptoms that are considered autoimmune.

A Slow but Steady Progression

HCV replicates and invades new cells at a slow rate. That's why it takes a long time to affect the health of the human being it lives in, accounting for the ten to thirty years that people carry the virus before developing symptoms.

The virus also continues to mutate once it is inside its host. This leads to a large degree of genetic variability in the virus. And genetic variability accounts for the high degree of resistance to antiviral therapy.

A person who has had hepatitis C for years can be expected to carry several variations of the original virus in his or her system. Antiviral therapy may be successful at killing several variations of the virus, but not all. It is not uncommon for a person to respond initially to antiviral therapy, but then, over time, a variant of the species replicates and symptoms return.

Facts about Transmission

It is almost impossible to be entirely free of the risk of contracting HCV. Global prevalence and the multitude of exposure routes make everyone vulnerable. However, exposure to HCV does not mean getting hepatitis C, and it is clear that some forms of exposure carry a higher risk of infection.

Blood-Borne Virus
A pathogenic virus that causes disease in humans and is found in the blood of infected individuals.

HCV is a blood-borne virus that is transmitted by virus-infected blood. Currently, approximately 20 percent of hepatitis C cases were contracted through blood transfusions. Starting in the early 1990s, transfusion agencies started screening potential donors and donated blood, largely eliminating this route of infection.

Blood transfusions are speculated to have elevated hepatitis C to epidemic proportions. For obvious reasons the origins of infected blood supplies is a sensitive topic. Thousands of hepatitis C patients received the disease unknowingly from blood banks and the manufacturers of blood products, and the potential for mass litigation is high.

Extensive global proliferation of HCV occurred during wars fought prior to modern blood-screening procedures. Many soldiers who received blood transfusions while overseas returned home and became blood donors. The virus traveled worldwide, undetected and invisible.

Transmission Through the Skin

Anytime the skin is punctured by an infected instrument, there is a risk of transmission. Intravenous (IV) drug use, vaccinations, dental procedures, tattoos, and piercings are examples. The most prevalent of these routes is IV drug use.

Currently, about 40 percent of hepatitis cases are thought to be the result of IV drug use. The tenacious nature of the virus makes it resistant to many disinfectant and sterilization techniques. HCV has survived up to three months in dried blood. Its tenacity allows it to withstand the sterilization techniques employed by IV drug users. It has been reported that many people contract the virus within the first year of IV drug use and as many as 30 percent from once-only experimentation.

IV drug use is the premier high-risk behavior. Anybody with a history of IV drug use, regardless of how they feel now, should be screened for hepatitis C.

A straight razor, acupuncture needle, vaccination needle, dental tool, tattoo instrument, and ear and body piercing instruments are all potential routes of transmission. Most professions that utilize these instruments have public-health measures in place to prevent the possibility of transmission. This is not true everywhere, and it's still unwise to get a back-alley tattoo in a faraway land.

Practically speaking, healthcare workers and those in other occupations with exposure to blood and tissue also are at risk of exposure. Needle-stick injuries account for about two percent of the hepatitis C population. Proper training protects the people in these occupations, but the sinister nature of the virus is still a threat.

Sexual Transmission

Hepatitis C can be transmitted sexually; however, sexual transmission is not the predominant route. Transmission is thought to occur via small abrasions and micro traumas that can occur during intercourse. Traumatic sexual activity and failure to use a condom are thought to increase the risk of transmission.

Transmission between low-risk monogamous sexual partners is low, but it's still important to take precautions. These precautions should be exercised outside the bedroom, as well. It's a good idea not to share items such as toothbrush, razor, nail clippers, and other instruments that may be exposed to small amounts of infected blood.

Theoretical Routes of Transmission

Several other routes of transmission are probable but have not been proven. Tropical-disease specialists were concerned about mosquitoes as a potential vector for hepatitis C. At this point this route is considered unlikely.

Vector
A carrier, particularly one that transmits disease.

It has been proposed that hepatitis C could be transmitted intranasally via sniffing cocaine. The idea is that specks of infected blood and mucus could be shared through the "rolled-up $20 bill" being passed around. This possibility has never been formally investigated.

There is one other alarming fact: In approximately 10 percent of patients, there is no identifiable cause for the disease. This is alarming because it suggests that all the potential routes of transmission are not fully understood.

Management of Hepatitis C

Successful management of hepatitis must be dynamic and able to change. A realistic goal for hepatitis C patients is to put the virus into remission and keep it there. Countermeasures to hepatitis C must be in place before liver damage becomes irreversible.

Conventional Medicine

The standard medical treatment for hepatitis C basically consists of two drugs: interferon and ribavirin. These drugs are expensive and associated with significant adverse side effects. To make matters worse, they appear to be minimally effective.

Few patients experience a cure from these drugs, and many experience the opposite. Patients taking medication for hepatitis can experience nausea, headache, fever, muscle pain, extreme fatigue, hair loss, irritability, depression, and lung and eye complications. And this is with only one of the drugs! When we add the second drug, the side effects of the combination therapy are considered "universal, significant, and possibly serious." This is further complicated by the fact that, at best, only about 50 percent of patients experience a lasting positive response after forty-eight weeks of feeling awful.

Orthodox medicine approaches hepatitis C from a reductionist model. Focus is on HCV and not on the patient. Many different laboratory tests are used to monitor viral replication while information on the patient's well-being is of secondary importance. Laboratory tests for hepatitis often do not correlate directly with how the patient feels. Doctors may dismiss patient complaints due to a lack of laboratory evidence. Many secondary symptoms of hepatitis are ignored because they cannot be explained.

Holistic practitioners focus on the patient's experience of the disease rather than on the disease itself. Subtle patterns of symptoms provide clues as to what a particular hepatitis patient may need. Acupuncture, chiropractic adjustment, herbs, vitamins, and other nutrients can be prescribed preventively. These treatments can prevent a crisis and the necessity for stronger pharmaceutical intervention.

Complementary and Alternative Medicine

Why would anyone with hepatitis consider using complementary and alternative medicine? The foundation of complementary and alternative medicine is the optimization of health through nutrition and lifestyle. Alternative practitioners understand that carrying HCV does not have to mean living with the disease.

One quarter of patients infected with HCV clear it without long-term effects. Currently, standard medical management for hepatitis recommends no treatment for HCV-positive patients without elevated liver enzymes. Why would you wait until the virus causes damage to act? The reason no treatment is recommended is that the drug therapies offered have a poor benefit-to-risk ratio. In fact, they can be downright dangerous. For patients in this position, it would be ludicrous to ignore nutritional, herbal, and lifestyle therapies that can prevent full-blown hepatitis.

The basic principles of complementary and alternative medicine strengthen any approach to hepatitis management. Historically, cleansing, fasting, and other forms of detoxification have provided a foundation for medical practices globally. The philosophy that, given the proper environment, the body has the power to heal itself and return to a normal healthy state, opens up new treatment options.

If treatment is limited to allopathic drug therapies, the body is not offered the optimal environment to defeat the virus and return to a healthy state. Water, exercise, vitamins, minerals, herbs, and other complementary and alternative therapies all support the detoxification process.

The primary reason that patients develop long-term hepatitis C may very well be the accumulation of unnecessary wastes that are not properly eliminated. Modern science has shown that many alternative treatments are safe and effective. It could be argued that ignoring the application of proven alternative therapies is a serious error of omission.

Another ironic aspect of hepatitis C is that if you carry the virus and feel lousy all the time but do not have abnormal lab tests, there is no treatment to recommend. Clearly, conventional medical doctors who treat hepatitis C have been pulling out their hair in frustration over this disease.

Necessity is the mother of invention. With so many millions of people afflicted with hepatitis C worldwide and so little that standard medical treatments have to offer, people have looked for alternatives. They have sought the help of medical practitioners of every discipline. Naturopaths, chiropractors, acupuncturists, osteopaths, Ayurvedic doctors, and many other healers have contributed valuable insights on new approaches to this emerging epidemic. Complementary and alternative practitioners have been successful in managing hepatitis C, leaving conventional doctors scratching their heads.

Finally, someone at the National Institutes of Health (NIH) got a bright idea. The clear need for inexpensive, nontoxic treatments for hepatitis C worldwide drove them to sponsor an international conference in 1999: "Complementary and Alternative Medicine in Chronic Liver Disease." Here, they brought together experts of different disciplines from all over the world. The goal of the NIH was to have an open mind to some of the "voodoo" being practiced out there by the different complementary and alternative medicine doctors. What they found was some legitimate medicine. Chapters 4 and 5 highlight some of the evidence-based alternative therapies that provide valuable treatment options to individuals who are HCV positive.

CHAPTER 4

DIET AND LIFESTYLE

The liver is a major component of the digestive system. Although no single diet is universally recommended for people suffering from hepatitis, certain accepted dietary excesses that facilitate the progression of the disease. This chapter discusses a commonsense diet that optimizes liver health and prevents the worsening of hepatitis symptoms.

Does Diet Really Affect Hepatitis?

The impact of diet on liver health is clearly documented in the film *Supersize Me*. Filmmaker Morgan Spurlock, in conjunction with a team of doctors, records the physiological impact of a thirty-day fast-food diet. In just one month Morgan develops elevated liver enzymes, fatty liver, and erectile dysfunction and gains twenty-two pounds.

The combined opinion of the cardiologist, internist, and general practitioner monitoring Morgan was that he had to stop the diet before his liver failed. In just two weeks Morgan's liver enzymes had gone from normal into the alarm range. No one was expecting liver damage to occur so quickly or to be so severe.

Other experiments have shown that obese children often have elevated liver enzymes. When researchers took liver samples from such children, the results were surprising. Fat accumulation, fibrosis, and scarring were evident in children's livers as early as age fifteen.

It has been speculated that having elevated liver enzymes as a child can reduce life expectancy by seventeen years. However, diet experts are often unwilling to make links between diet and disease. It becomes the job of crusaders, such as filmmaker Morgan Spurlock, to open up the dialog about the potential problem.

The SAD Diet

The standard American diet is commonly referred to as the "SAD" diet. The liver will be the first to tell you why. The SAD diet is high in processed foods that are full of preservatives, coloring agents, sweeteners, and oils. These compounds are created in food-science laboratories for the sole purpose of making food cost less, last longer, and look prettier.

A great example of this is the hydrogenation of oils to create margarine or shortening. This process includes mixing inexpensive (and probably rancid) oil with nickel oxide, subjecting it to hydrogen gas, bleaching out the gray color, dyeing it, and adding a synthetic flavoring agent. Is this still food?

What scientists did not realize is that the chemical changes that occur during these processes resulted in a *trans*-fat, which turns out to be toxic to the body. These hydrogenated oils wreak havoc on cellular metabolism, especially in the liver.

Rest assured, the Food and Drug Administration (FDA) is taking care of the matter. By January 2006 all packaged food products are required to list the trans-fatty-acid content of processed food on the label.

This pressures food companies to replace trans-fatty acids before they have to reveal their dirty little secrets. Ironically, potential solutions include genetically engineered soybeans that supposedly create oils with favorable fatty-acid profiles. These synthetic solutions are sure to create new and greater challenges for liver metabolism.

So What Do I Eat?

There is no gold standard when it comes to diet recommendations for hepatitis. The different stages of hepatitis infection have different fluid and nutritional requirements. An acute flare-up requires fluids, electrolytes, and easily digested foods, while chronic inactive hepatitis needs adequate nutritional building blocks for cell repair and regeneration.

The best approach consists of merging the available scientific evidence with old-fashioned common sense. Dieticians are often responsible for delivering science-based dietary treatments. Dieticians "prescribe diets" that can be overwhelmingly associated with numbers, ratios, and percentages. When diet advice comes in the form of total number of calories, grams of fat, protein, carbohydrates, and fiber, and glycemic index, it can be overwhelming. The numbers game provides a scientific foundation for diet recommendations, but it can become impractical.

However, we do need to spell out important diet numbers that are recommended for hepatitis patients. The average 150-pound adult who is positive for the hepatitis C virus should eat 2,000–2,500 calories daily. This should include 70–100 grams of protein (except in advanced cirrhosis).

Protein is particularly important. It is necessary for liver regeneration and to support ammonia detoxification. The ideal is to have as much of this protein as possible come from vegetable sources. If appetite and weight loss are problematic, a good-quality protein powder (whey or rice) can be used to supplement the diet.

Approximately 60 grams, or 20 to 30 percent of daily calories, should be derived from fat. The majority of dietary fat should be good fat, such as mono- and polyunsaturated fatty acids (PUFAs). It is important to minimize saturated and trans-fatty-acid intake.

PUFA
The fatty acid that makes up polyunsaturated fats, which are liquid at room temperature.

In 1995, *The American Journal of Epidemiology* published a study showing that high-fat diets coupled with reduced protein and carbohydrates increased the risk of hepatitis C progressing to cirrhosis. This makes total sense. Combine Morgan Spurlock's thirty-day fast-food diet with the HCV, and of course it increases the risk of progression.

A low-fat diet that includes cold-pressed oils, nuts, seeds, and cold-water fish has an anti-inflammatory effect on the liver in chronic hepatitis. The omega-3 fatty acids found in cold-water fish serve as functional foods by providing nutritional, as well as anti-inflammatory, activity. Hepatitis patients should consume 4 grams daily of omega-3 fatty acids, which can come from combined diet and supplemental sources.

The Commonsense Approach

There is no ideal diet for everyone. Regardless of hepatitis infection, the ideal diet is individualized and must be able to fluctuate with our needs. Diet should vary with activity level, state of health, where we live, time of year, and even daily weather.

The commonsense diet is a whole-foods diet based on lean meat, poultry, dairy, vegetables, fruit, and grain. The dietician's numbers serve as a guideline for creating the relative proportions of the whole foods to be eaten in the commonsense diet.

Diet should be a high priority for hepatitis patients. The goal is to nourish the body and provide the best possible chance for optimum energy, immune function, and cellular repair. Simply putting calories in our mouths to get by isn't good enough.

To manage hepatitis, the diet should be flexible, natural, balanced, and moderate. It should be based on whole grains, legumes, abundant vegetables, lean meats, dairy, nuts, seeds, and fruit. Notice, none of these foods is processed.

To put these diet recommendations into action, you need to:

- Eat five or more servings a day of vegetables and fruit.

- Eat four servings of starchy plants, such as squash, beans, and whole grains.

- Have three servings a day of protein, such as nuts, seeds, fish, eggs, poultry, lamb, beef, wild game, and pork.

- Eat two servings of milk, cheese, and yogurt, if tolerated.

The mealtime ritual is important. Meals should be eaten sitting down in a relaxed atmosphere. Studies have shown that the first enzymatic steps of digestion occur when we smell our food. Proper mental focus on chewing and enjoying our meal prepares the liver for its upcoming metabolic duties.

Hepatitis patients need to avoid caffeine, alcohol, fried and fatty foods, oxidized and synthetic fatty acids, synthetic sweeteners and sugar, additives, preservatives, and coloring agents. All these foods lack nutritional value and put stress on the liver.

A Lifestyle That Detoxifies

There are several no-brainer lifestyle choices that absolutely cannot be ignored. Any person, regardless of health status, should follow these guidelines. Following these recommendations decreases exposure to unnecessary toxins.

First and foremost, if you are HCV positive, do not smoke or drink alcohol. Eliminate recreational drug use, and minimize or eliminate caffeine. These basic steps eliminate major toxins that can destroy the liver, even in the absence of viral disease.

Soda is a popular toxin that is ingested by millions of people worldwide. Some people drink soda in place of water. This is equivalent to poisoning yourself slowly. There is no specific link between soda consumption and the progression of hepatitis C, but consider the following facts:

- You can put a steak in a bowl of soda, and it will dissolve in two days.

- Soda is used to remove rust spots from chrome car bumpers.

- Pour a can of soda over dirty battery terminals, and it will bubble away the corrosion.

- The active ingredient in soda is phosphoric acid, which can dissolve a nail in four days.

- A certain soda manufacturer has been using its soda to clean the engines of its trucks for more than thirty years.

The choice to take a prescription medication should be an informed choice, making sure to avoid unnecessary medications. Talk to a doctor or pharmacist about the benefit versus risk of all prescription and over-the-counter medications. If you have a condition that can possibly be managed without medication, do so.

Many of the changes you will make to manage hepatitis will have a positive impact on other disease conditions. Conditions such as hypertension and high cholesterol may correct themselves through diet and lifestyle changes. Choose a doctor who will support your goal of reducing prescription medicines to those that are absolutely necessary.

If your doctor understands the complexity and unpredictability of hepatitis, he or she should appreciate your dedication to treating your liver well. You and your doctor can set reasonable goals to wean yourself from unnecessary medications. This can be challenging, but it could mean the difference between a healthy functioning liver and being on a transplant list.

Support from Other Organs of Detoxification

Apart from killing the virus, the goal for hepatitis C management includes aiding the liver in its many detoxification functions. The majority of treatments discussed in this book aim to reduce the total toxic load taken into the body or directly aid the liver in detoxification. We have yet to discuss how other organs of detoxification can help take some of the workload off the liver.

The body has multiple channels of elimination for toxins. Toxins can be eliminated through the stool, urine, skin, and breath. To avoid toxin overload, it's important to keep all channels of elimination open and functioning optimally.

Move Toxins Out with the Stool

Toxins that have been metabolized by the liver are eliminated through the stool. Constipation causes the stool to remain in the bowels for extended periods of time. This allows toxins to be reabsorbed from the stool into the body. All efforts should be made to stay "regular," having a minimum of one bowel movement daily. Ideally, there should be a bowel movement for each meal eaten. If constipation occurs, taking a high-quality fiber supplement can correct the problem.

Fiber supplements such as psyllium-seed powder, apple pectin, and prune powder create bulking action in the stool and promote normal bowel health. They facilitate the drawing out of stored toxins and enhance intestinal elimination of toxins released into the stool.

Eliminate Wastes through the Skin

The skin is the largest organ of elimination. Toxins are released when we sweat, shed skin cells, and cut our hair and nails, as well as through oil glands in the skin. Sweat contains uric acid, electrolytes, and other water-soluble waste products. Oil glands secrete fat-soluble waste products similar to those excreted from the liver into the bile.

The sweat and oil secretions of people undergoing detoxification have been found to contain a variety of toxic substances that they had been previously exposed to. Substances that can be released through the skin include nicotine, tar, anesthetics, pesticides, heavy metals, and other chemicals.

Quality nutrition and plenty of clean water are the foundations of healthy skin. Increased sweating through exercise and saunas can promote toxin release. In addition, increasing circulation to the skin enhances this important elimination route.

Dry-skin brushing is a natural-medicine technique that promotes increased circulation to the skin and the shedding of dead skin cells, dried sweat, and microscopic debris. Dry-skin brushing is done using a natural-bristle brush or a loofah sponge. Stand naked before showering and gently brush the skin from the tips of the arms and legs along all surfaces of the body toward the heart.

The use of dry-skin brushing dates back thousands of years. It is gentle, effective, and free! Don't underestimate the impact that this simple procedure, when done daily, can have on reducing the body's total toxin load.

Breathe Away the Toxins

The lungs eliminate gas and vapors from the body. Their primary job is to excrete carbon dioxide, a waste product of cellular metabolism. This process maintains the correct acid/base balance, which is necessary for the regulation of homeostasis.

Homeostasis
Maintenance of the internal environment of the body, naturally preserved by adaptive responses that promote healthy survival.

The lungs are involved in elimination, as well as absorption. If the gas-exchange surface of the lung responsible for absorbing oxygen is spread out, it's as big as a tennis court! This surface is only a few cell layers thick, leaving it vulnerable to the absorption of unwanted air pollution, as well.

Healthy lungs are hydrated and breathe fresh oxygenated air fully and deeply. Breathing exercises and stimulating physical exercise increase respiratory rate and depth. Daily deep breathing is an important component of eliminating unwanted toxins from the body.

Breathing exercises can be done anywhere and anytime. Sit comfortably, and take long, deep, slow breaths through the nostrils. Allow the breath to be gentle and relaxed as you slightly contract the back of your throat creating a steady hissing sound as you breathe in and out. Lengthen the time of the inhalation and exhalation as much as possible without creating tension anywhere in your body. That's all there is to it.

Eliminate as You Urinate

The kidneys continuously filter toxins from the blood, eliminate products broken down from the cells, and delicately balance the electrolytes and water. Water makes up the majority of our body. It facilitates the chemical reactions that take place inside the cells and carries nutrients, chemicals, and oxygen to the cells while collecting cellular secretions and waste for transport and elimination.

It's essential to drink plenty of clean water to assist the complete removal of toxins through the kidneys. It is recommended that the number of ounces of water you consume daily equals half the number of pounds of your body weight. For example, if your body weight is 160 pounds, your water intake should be 80 ounces daily.

The influence of water on chronic disease is entirely underestimated. Approximately 75 percent of Americans are chronically dehydrated. It has been estimated that drinking five glasses of water daily decreases the risk of colon cancer by 45 percent, breast cancer by 79 percent, and bladder cancer by 50 percent. Even mild dehydration has been shown to trigger fatigue, fuzzy short-term memory, focusing difficulty, and slower metabolism.

Drinking adequate water is a basic necessity for general health maintenance and detoxification. And it's important to remember that there are no substitutes for water. Tea, coffee, and soda do the opposite of hydrating our tissues.

It is important to drink the purest water available to you. Bottled, filtered, and spring water are the best choices. Carry a full water bottle with you to work or school to ensure access to plenty of water throughout the day.

If you are unaccustomed to drinking adequate water, during the first few days it will seem like too much. You will find yourself urinating frequently, and your urine will be clear, colorless, and odorless. Think of a dry sponge on which water is poured. Initially, the water just runs off the surface. Gradually, the sponge begins to absorb the water until it is saturated. At this point, excess water just trickles out the bottom of the sponge. A similar process will happen to you.

Keep the Lymphatic System Moving

The lymphatic system carries lymph throughout the body. Lymph comes from the fluid that surrounds and bathes the cells, bringing in nourishment and removing waste. Lymph travels in the lymphatic vessels, which lie right next to the blood vessels and eventually connect back to the major veins.

Lymph
A clear fluid that contains immune cells, proteins, waste, and other elements, circulating throughout the lymphatic vessels.

The lymph nodes are positioned along the lymph vessels and contain a high concentration of immune cells that engulf and break down potentially toxic substances. Lymph nodes act as mini livers, capable of detoxifying bacteria, viruses, and toxins. These nodes enlarge at times when they go into action, such as during an infection.

Unlike the vascular system, the lymphatic system does not have the luxury of the heart to pump it along. The lymph relies on the contraction of the surrounding muscles. A sedentary lifestyle allows lymph to stagnate and toxins to build up. Regular stretching, exercise, and massage all move the muscles in a way that stimulates the lymph to move.

Castor-oil packs are a therapy from antiquity that provides excellent movement of the lymph fluid. Castor oil taken internally is used as a powerful cathartic laxative that stimulates the bowel to evacuate. It is so potent that when applied topically, it causes the lymph vessels to gently pump lymph fluid.

The digestive system is closely linked to the lymphatic system for obvious reasons. The gut-associated lymphatic tissue, known as GALT, is the first line of defense against invading toxins taken in through the mouth. Castor-oil packs applied to the abdomen stimulate GALT and prevent lymph stagnation.

To make a castor-oil pack, you need a piece of cotton flannel, castor oil, a hand towel, and a heating pad or hot-water bottle. Apply castor oil to the cotton flannel, and place it over the abdomen, making sure it covers the liver. A dry towel is placed over the pack, and heat is applied over the towel. Leave the pack in place for forty-five minutes.

Ten Lifestyle Tips That Support Liver Health

Diet and lifestyle have a major impact on health and wellness. For individuals who are positive for HCV, a good diet and lifestyle can make all the difference in quality of life. This chapter has covered some simple, valuable, and inexpensive ways to take charge of some of the disease factors within your control.

1. Avoid coffee.

2. Avoid alcohol.

3. Avoid soda.

4. Avoid recreational drugs.

5. Minimize prescription medications.

6. Drink enough water.

7. Exercise regularly; this should include deep breathing and sweating.

8. Eat a whole-foods diet that includes high-quality protein, omega-3 fats, vegetables, fruit, and whole grains.

9. Practice dry-skin brushing daily.

10. Use castor-oil packs regularly.

CHAPTER 5

VITAMINS, MINERALS, AND OTHER NUTRIENTS

The health of an individual with hepatitis determines how affected he or she will be by it. The correct nutritional and detoxifying supplements can prevent the onset or recurrence of debilitating hepatitis symptoms. This chapter highlights the vitamins, minerals, and other nutritional substances helpful in managing hepatitis.

Vitamin E

Vitamin E is the ultimate fat-soluble free-radical scavenger, a molecule that binds to free electrons, resulting in the neutralization of a potentially damaging compound. Vitamin E is also known for its immune-enhancing and anti-inflammatory activity. To the surprise of many vitamin skeptics, vitamin E deficiency is relatively common in the developed world.

Let's look at vitamin E's potential value to individuals with hepatitis. First, as a free-radical scavenger, it squelches the free radicals created by damaged cells before they do further damage. Second, vitamin E reduces liver inflammation. Third, vitamin E can enhance the immune response, helping to kill off the hepatitis virus.

Several studies have successfully used vitamin E, at doses in the range 400–1,200 international units (IU) daily, to treat hepatitis. One study showed that vitamin E reduced liver enzymes in patients who did not respond to interferon therapy. A different study showed that vitamin E enhanced the outcome of interferon therapy.

When considering vitamin E supplements, always look for naturally occurring d-alpha-tocopherol or mixed-tocopherol supplements. The safe, daily, upper-intake level of vitamin E is set at 1,000 IU, and hepatitis patients should consider taking 800 IU daily. However, vitamin E does have a mild blood-thinning effect, so you should consult your healthcare professional before taking it.

N-Acetyl Cysteine

Throughout this book I have stressed the importance of glutathione. Glutathione levels are critical to defend all cells from damaging free radicals. Hepatitis patients are at particular risk for losing the support of this vital compound.

N-acetyl cysteine is a modified form of the dietary amino acid cysteine, which serves as a precursor to glutathione synthesis. For this reason N-acetyl cysteine is a valuable therapeutic agent in the treatment of cancer, heart disease, heavy-metal toxicity, and other diseases characterized by oxidative damage.

When taken orally, N-acetyl cysteine is rapidly absorbed into the body and has been shown to be an effective method for increasing glutathione biosynthesis. The bottom line is: N-acetyl cysteine promotes glutathione synthesis and increases glutathione levels in the body.

The most well-known use of N-acetyl cysteine is as an antidote to acetaminophen (Tylenol) poisoning. Acetaminophen depletes the liver of glutathione and, in large doses, can cause liver damage and even death. If N-acetyl cysteine is given within twenty-four hours of an overdose, it can save lives—and livers.

Studies using N-acetyl cysteine to treat hepatitis C are limited to a combined treatment with interferon. Often patients can be resistant to interferon therapy or develop a resistance over time. N-acetyl cysteine can change that.

Taking 600 milligrams (mg) of N-acetyl cysteine for six months enhanced the response of interferon therapy in chronic hepatitis-C patients who were resistant to interferon. This is great news! Significant decreases were seen in liver enzymes and measurements of viral activity.

The media is always quick to point out negative or potentially dangerous drug/nutrient interactions, an example being the over-publicized risk of increased bleeding when vitamin E is taken with blood-thinning medication. Rarely do we see positive drug/nutrient interactions such as N-acetyl cysteine and interferon, and N-acetyl cysteine protecting the liver from acetaminophen.

N-acetyl cysteine is generally safe and well-tolerated, even at high doses. Typical doses for N-acetyl cysteine range from 600–1,800 mg daily. Hepatitis C studies have utilized 600 mg three times a day in conjunction with interferon. More research is necessary to explore the full potential of N-acetyl cysteine individually or in combination with other nutrients and herbs to treat hepatitis.

Phosphatidyl Choline

Phosphatidyl choline is the predominant nutrient found in all the cell membranes in the body. It serves as an important reservoir for choline, a B vitamin that is required for proper functioning of the nervous system, liver, and gallbladder. Phosphatidyl choline has been used for many kinds of liver problems, including hepatitis and cirrhosis.

Phosphatidyl choline helps with general body detoxification by aiding in fat emulsification, transport, and utilization. This decongests the liver of the excess fat and toxins that have accumulated.

This nutrient has also been documented to aid in the repair of liver damage. After damage to liver cells, substantial replacement of cell membranes occurs. Phosphatidyl choline is a necessary component of each of the replaced membranes.

More than eight double-blind trials and other biochemical experiments have shown that phosphatidyl choline has a clinical benefit in cases of liver damage. It has been shown to reduce liver enzymes, restore well-being, and improve overall survival from chronic liver disease.

A multicenter double-blind human trial published in *Hepatogastroenterology* showed that phosphatidyl choline given after twenty-four weeks of interferon resulted in a longer term of improvement than interferon alone. Some scientists feel that phosphatidyl choline may be a breakthrough in the nutritional management of hepatitis C.

There are no known toxic effects from phosphatidyl choline, even at very high doses. Practitioners use dosages of phosphatidyl choline in the range of 1–15 grams daily. Clinical research done on hepatitis patients used 1,500–2,000 mg daily.

Phosphatidyl choline is available by itself in a capsule, or it can be found in lecithin, a popular food source for this valuable nutrient. Be aware that lecithin includes from 10 to 20 percent phosphatidyl choline. Lecithin can be used as a source of phosphatidyl choline, but the dose must be adjusted.

Fish Oils

Essential Fatty Acids
Fatty acids that are not manufactured by the body and must be obtained from the diet.

You would have to live in a hole not to have heard about the many health benefits of omega-3 fatty acids found in fish oil. In 2002 the U.S. Surgeon General declared that about 70 percent of chronic disease is related to an imbalance or excess of fatty acids in the diet. So many diets worldwide are deficient in the essential omega-3 fatty acids eicosapentaenoic acid (EPA) and docosahexaenoic acid (DHA).

Omega-3 fatty acids are precursors of eicosanoids, compounds that regulate inflammation. Without proper eicosanoid production, inflammation can run rampant in the body. Individuals with hepatitis want to do everything they can to reduce inflammation.

Eicosanoids
A family of compounds that regulate pain and swelling, help maintain blood-pressure and cholesterol levels, and promote nerve-impulse transmission.

In addition to being valuable anti-inflammatory agents, EPA and DHA have been shown to have anti–hepatitis C activity. This makes fish oil the perfect complement to any hepatitis C protocol. Naturopathic physician Bruce Millman, N.D., associate professor at Bastyr University in Seattle, recommends two teaspoons daily of a high-quality cod-liver oil for his hepatitis patients.

Cod-Liver Oil
Oil from the liver of cod that contains small amounts of naturally occurring vitamins A, D, and E.

A Note about Cod-Liver-Oil Safety

Not all cod-liver oil is created equal. Unfortunately, our oceans are not immune to the toxic environment we have created. Toxins such as mercury, lead, PCBs, and dioxins are released into the environment in alarming proportions. These toxins accumulate in fish and other wildlife.

A high-quality fish-oil product must be molecularly distilled to remove environmental contaminants. Once distilled, the results of laboratory tests to verify that these toxins have been removed should be available from the fish-oil manufacturer. If this information is not readily available, ask for it!

Cod-liver oil contains small amounts of naturally occurring vitamins A, D, and E. It is important not to consume excess quantities of these fat-soluble vitamins. The small, naturally occurring amounts of these vitamins in cod-liver oil do not pose a threat of overdoing it. However, some manufacturers add larger amounts of these vitamins to their products. Be sure to add up all the vitamins A, D, and E being consumed in your nutritional program (considering the particular brands you choose), and follow the recommended amounts for these three nutrients.

Whey Protein

Adequate dietary protein is necessary for liver-cell regeneration. Hepatitis patients should be eating 70–100 grams of high-quality, low-fat protein daily. The best source of protein for hepatitis patients is vegetable protein. Eating 70–100 grams of vegetable protein daily is hard for even the most dedicated patient. Other sources of animal meats and dairy are valuable, but they are also high in saturated fat.

A good-quality protein powder can be used as a supplement. Whey protein supplies a complete and easily assimilated low-fat protein. In addition, whey contains high amounts of biological components that have been shown to be immune-enhancing and antiviral and to scavenge free radicals.

Biologic Activity of Whey Protein

Whey is considered a functional food with a number of health benefits beyond its basic nutritional profile. Whey is naturally rich in lactoferrin and other immune-system proteins that have huge potential in the nutritional management of hepatitis C.

Functional Food

A food with medicinal qualities that go beyond its basic nutritional content.

Lactoferrin is a protein released into human secretions such as mucus, tears, sweat, and breast milk. It serves as a first line of defense against invading viruses and bacteria. When these microorganisms are detected, lactoferrin binds the nutrients surrounding the invader and starves it out.

In addition to being a valuable antimicrobial, whey protein is a potent antioxidant. Whey is rich in the amino acid cysteine, which is the precursor to glutathione, the most potent intracellular antioxidant in the body.

Lactoferrin
A biologically active protein that is found in human bodily secretions and is anti-inflammatory, antimicrobial, and immune-enhancing.

Glutathione is a naturally occurring protective molecule found in all human cells. It is the main antioxidant in hepatic tissue and in all mammalian tissues. When cells become depleted of glutathione, they die. The clinical relevance of glutathione's applications has interested researchers for decades. However, the bioavailability of glutathione supplements has been disappointing. Whey-protein supplementation is one of the few ways shown to raise cellular glutathione levels.

Scientific evidence shows that chronic liver diseases, including hepatitis, deplete cellular glutathione levels. *In vitro* studies have shown that the biological components of whey prevent the hepatitis C virus (HCV) from infecting human liver cells. Studies on humans indicate that whey is an effective, nontoxic, and low-fat protein with valuable antiviral and antioxidant activity.

There have been no large-scale double-blind trials to determine the optimal dose, duration of treatment, or potential effects of combining whey with the pharmaceutical management of hepatitis C. Whey proteins are processed in a variety of ways for different applications. Unhydrolyzed whey proteins contain the highest amount of antiviral and immune-enhancing potential.

An appropriate dose of whey protein for hepatitis patients is based on the protein content in the diet. The combination of dietary protein and whey should be 70–100 grams. For many adults, this works out to approximately 12–15 grams of whey protein daily.

Antioxidants in the Treatment of Hepatitis C

Liver cirrhosis is the result of fibrosis and scarring within liver cells. Our discussion of basic liver structure revealed that the liver is highly concentrated with cell membranes. Recent evidence has shown that free-radical damage to liver-cell membranes is a unifying mechanism underlying liver destruction in all types of chronic liver disease.

Cell destruction occurs in an environment that is high in free radicals and low in antioxidants. This is a natural process that results from the interactions between immune cells and invading toxins or viruses. When HCV interacts with hepatic immune cells, large amounts of free radicals are released into the surrounding tissue. If the free radicals generated do not meet antioxidants, cellular dysfunction begins. Cells begin to lose shape and function and are slowly replaced by fibers and scars.

The bottom line is: Supplementing the diet with antioxidants protects liver cells. The problem is that there are so many antioxidant supplements to choose from. Luckily, there are a few key antioxidants that have been found to be particularly important in the treatment of hepatitis.

Alpha-Lipoic Acid

Alpha-lipoic acid has been labeled the universal antioxidant. It is considered "universal" because it exhibits potent free-radical scavenging activity in both the watery and fatty compartments of the cell. Other valuable antioxidants, such as vitamin C (water-soluble) and vitamin E (fat-soluble), work only in one environment or the other.

Research has shown that alpha-lipoic acid neutralizes dangerous free radicals that play a role in the development of chronic diseases, including atherosclerosis, lung disease, chronic inflammation, and neurological disorders. Alpha-lipoic acid also acts as a synergist with other antioxidants in the body by recycling and extending the life span of vitamin C, glutathione, and vitamin E.

Few other antioxidants can provide the versatile protection offered by alpha-lipoic acid. It fulfills the requirements of a valuable therapeutic supplement by being readily absorbed and easily converted to a usable form. It also has a variety of antioxidant actions and is active in all the compartments of the cell.

Providing the body with more antioxidants than free radicals prevents hepatitis from damaging cells and tissue, slowing the progression of the disease. As you can see, alpha-lipoic acid is potentially a highly effective therapeutic agent for hepatitis.

Alpha-lipoic acid was only discovered in the 1950s, and researchers did not really begin to understand its value until the early 1980s. The therapeutic impact of alpha-lipoic acid on hepatitis C is just beginning to be explored in a clinical setting.

Burt Berkson, M.D., Ph.D., director of the Integrative Medical Center of New Mexico in Las Cruces, has done a lot of clinical work on hepatitis C. He has published several case reports that begin to shed light on the value of alpha-lipoic acid in treating hepatitis C.

Dr. Berkson has developed a low-cost and effective "triple-antioxidant" treatment strategy. He combines alpha-lipoic acid, milk thistle, and selenium for their free-radical-quenching, antiviral, and immune-boosting properties. In a 1999 publication, he described the effect of triple-antioxidant therapy on three patients with cirrhosis, portal hypertension, and esophageal varices secondary to chronic HCV infection.

The patients all showed remarkable improvements in symptoms and laboratory values. At the time of publication, all three patients were reported to be back at work, carrying out their normal activities, and feeling healthy. Most important, liver transplants were avoided. One year of the triple-antioxidant therapy costs $2,000 compared to approximately $300,000 for a transplant. It is clearly reasonable from both a financial and a therapeutic viewpoint to begin less invasive nutritional interventions before liver damage is so severe that a transplant is necessary.

We must also give credit to pioneers, such as Dr. Berkson, for researching and publishing such valuable data. Case studies with positive outcomes prompt larger clinical trials to be performed. Hopefully, researchers will continue to explore the value of antioxidant therapies, such as alpha-lipoic acid, to treat chronic hepatitis C.

Oligomeric Proanthocyanidin Complexes (OPCs)

OPCs are a powerful group of antioxidants found in numerous plant and food sources. They are particularly useful for protecting small blood vessels and capillaries from oxidative damage. In addition to antioxidant activity, OPCs serve as guardians against other substances that degrade the structure of the blood vessels.

As we age, our blood vessels come under attack. They lose their structural integrity and become leaky. Varicose veins, hemorrhoids, and swollen ankles are examples of what happens when vessels become leaky. OPCs can come to the rescue of the many small blood vessels in the liver. When hepatitis progresses to cirrhosis, blood vessels become fragile. Veins and capillaries can lose their ability to function, resulting in multiple problems.

An eight-week, double-blind, placebo-controlled study using OPCs for patients with cirrhosis showed significantly improved capillary strength. The great thing about OPCs is that when they are not busy protecting capillaries, they can be aggressively scavenging free radicals. In a nutshell, OPCs provide double protection against hepatitis and its damaging forces at work in the liver.

More Is Not Always Better

It is important to recognize that taking more of a supplement is not always a good idea. Here are some nutrients available in supplement form that you should be cautious about.

Iron

Iron deficiency is the most common nutrient deficiency in the world. Groups at high risk are children, menstruating women, pregnant women, and the elderly. However, excess iron supplementation can be harmful.

Iron in excess acts as a dangerous free radical. Hepatitis patients constantly struggle to keep more antioxidants than free radicals available. They cannot afford any additional free radicals, such as excess iron, roaming around waiting to do cell damage.

Hepatitis patients who develop liver cancer have been found to have excess concentrations of iron deposits in their liver cells. It is thought that excess iron in the liver encourages liver cells to mutate and become cancerous.

Dietary iron should be the sole source of iron for hepatitis patients. Supplemental iron should be avoided unless there is laboratory evidence of an iron deficiency.

Vitamin A

Another vitamin to keep an eye on is vitamin A. This vitamin is fat-soluble and is stored in the liver.

Hypervitaminosis can occur with excess vitamin A intake. Too much vitamin A can cause loss of appetite, hair loss, dry skin, headaches, and nausea.

> **Hyper-vitaminosis**
> A condition resulting from excessive intake of toxic amounts of one or more vitamins, especially over a long period of time.

The flip side here is that vitamin A is a powerful immune-boosting vitamin. It supports cell division and is known to protect the body against cancer. Doesn't this sound like something hepatitis C patients need? Vitamin A is not something you want to avoid altogether. To avoid too much vitamin A, take no more than 25,000 IU daily.

Sometimes, vitamin A–supplement labels can be confusing. Vitamin A comes in more than one form. Beta-carotene is a vitamin A precursor that is labeled as vitamin A. The good news is that the beta-carotene form of vitamin A is not as stressful on the liver.

An extra-safe approach to vitamin A supplementation is to limit straight vitamin A consumption to 2,500 IU. The remaining vitamin A can be taken as beta-carotene.

Vitamin D

Vitamin D is a fat-soluble vitamin that is available in the diet and manufactured by the body. The body makes vitamin D when the skin is exposed to sunlight. Supplemental vitamin D has been shown to have therapeutic benefit in conditions such as osteoporosis, diabetes, and hypertension.

When vitamin D is consumed in considerable excess, it can cause symptoms of toxicity. The current maximum safe daily intake is set at 2,000 IU daily. However, the dose at which vitamin D becomes toxic is a matter of dispute. What we do know is that if toxic levels of vitamin D are consumed, they will contribute to liver damage. Chronic liver disease theoretically lowers the amount of vitamin D needed to cause adverse symptoms.

It is not completely clear how concerned HCV positive individuals should be about supplemental vitamin D intake. However, it is important to add together all the supplemental vitamin D being taken. The total amount of dietary and supplemental vitamin D should not exceed 2,000 IU daily.

What about a Multivitamin?

The body maintains health and vitality via thousands of enzymes. Vitamins and minerals serve as cofactors to enzyme function. Although many vitamins have not been specifically studied for the treatment of hepatitis C, they are still essential for total body health.

The multisystem effects of hepatitis C make it clear that liver protection is not the only goal for optimal management of the condition. Let's look at how some other vitamins and minerals might help a hepatitis C patient.

A high-quality multivitamin should contain all of the B vitamin family. B vitamins support the liver's cytochrome P-450 enzyme system. We already know how important cytochrome P-450 is for phase one liver detoxification. In addition, B vitamins also play a role in immune function and energy. People taking B vitamins will often report increased energy or a "pick-me-up" effect. This is because B vitamins support adrenal function, which is responsible for maintaining energy.

A good multivitamin should also contain vitamin C. It is a water-soluble antioxidant with a wide range of health benefits. Vitamin C is an essential nutrient for overall health and immune-system function.

Nobel Prize laureate Linus Pauling advocated vitamin C as a powerful therapy by itself. He believed that megadoses of vitamin C could provide antiviral activity capable of eliminating viruses such as HCV. Megadosing of vitamin C has not been shown to be effective for hepatitis C. However, taking a few grams of supplemental vitamin C daily provides additional free-radical-scavenging power to the body.

We could discuss every vitamin and mineral in a multivitamin and how it helps liver function, but that would be a book in itself. The bottom line is: A multivitamin is good nutritional insurance. When dietary intake fluctuates, you can be sure that the basic vitamins and minerals will be there to serve the liver.

There are a couple of other important things to consider when choosing a multivitamin. First, unless you have a verified iron deficiency, get a multivitamin without iron. Second, choose a multivitamin with 12,500–25,000 IU vitamin A (2,500 IU from vitamin A palmitate and the rest from beta-carotene).

High-quality multivitamins usually need to be taken more than once a day. More ingredients do not equate to a better vitamin. Choose a multivitamin that is limited to vitamins and minerals, avoiding brands with many additional nutritional compounds. We want to be pretty specific about the other nutritional and herbal medicines that will benefit the liver.

CHAPTER 6

HERBS THAT
BENEFIT THE LIVER

The lack of safe and effective drug treatments for hepatitis C has kept scientists searching for alternatives. Traditional liver-protecting herbs that have been used for thousands of years are beginning to be validated by research. This chapter covers several herbs that have been shown to be safe and effective in the management of hepatitis C.

Primitive Discoveries for Liver Protection

The origin of medicine stems from ancient times, when our ancestors chewed on roots and leaves to cure their ailments. However, the focus of modern medicine has moved away from herbs. Instead, we rely on synthetic drugs to find a cure for what ails us.

Ironically, modern research has rekindled an interest in herbal medicine. Numerous scientific studies have demonstrated the health-promoting effects of various plants. In some situations, herbs have been found to be superior to and safer than their synthetic counterparts.

Liver-protecting herbs were important to early civilizations. Humans were constantly searching for and sampling new plants to satisfy their appetites. Some unfortunate individuals discovered poisonous plants instead of food. The results were probably fatal. However, these resourceful civilizations quickly found herbs to provide antidotes to poisonings. What they did not realize was that they had discovered medicines that are effective against liver disease—a task that modern medicine is still fumbling through. Researchers have realized that taking a closer look at our ancestors' discoveries is not such a bad idea.

Milk Thistle

The milk-thistle plant, *Silybum marianum*, has been used in the treatment of poisonings and other liver conditions for more than 2,000 years. It is considered one of the oldest known herbal medicines. With more than 450 published studies using milk thistle to treat liver disease, it is one of the most potent and well-known liver-protecting plants that we know.

Milk thistle protects the liver in three ways. First, it directly acts as a guardian for liver cells by blocking the entrance of toxins and poisons. Second, it is a potent free-radical scavenger. And third, milk thistle has the ability to regenerate liver cells when they have been damaged or destroyed.

Milk Thistle as a Liver-Cell Guardian

Early experimental studies of milk thistle were done while investigating the deadly toxins found in the poisonous mushroom *Amanita phalloides*. Ingesting this mushroom causes swift, severe, and often fatal damage to liver cells. It was discovered that milk thistle has the ability to bind the outside of the liver cells and block the entrance of the deadly toxin. In addition, it was found that milk thistle enables the neutralization of any toxins that have already entered the cells.

In animal studies, it has been demonstrated that milk thistle given ten minutes after ingesting *Amanita phalloides* toxin completely counteracted the toxic effects. When given within twenty-four hours, it prevented death and greatly reduced liver damage.

The mechanism of liver damage in hepatitis C patients is not totally understood. On one hand, we know that HCV is directly toxic to liver cells. On the other hand, we know that the body creates compounds in response to the virus that are also toxic the liver.

One thing that is clear is that when milk thistle binds to the outside of liver cells and acts as a guardian, a hepatitis C patient is much better off. Multiple studies have shown that milk thistle can speed recovery from acute hepatitis. Other studies have shown that milk thistle aids in the reduction of symptoms associated with chronic hepatitis and can return elevated liver enzymes to normal.

Milk Thistle as a Free-Radical Scavenger

HCV is cytopathic and damages hepatocytes directly. It is also immunopathic, which means that it can cause an immune response that is responsible for damaging the liver. The normally small and inconspicuous Kupffer's cells undergo enlargement and proliferation. If HCV lingers and the Kupffer's cells are forced to recruit other immune-system cells to the area for an all-out war, the liver becomes a battleground between the immune system and the virus.

As the battle rages, free radicals are generated within the liver. To make matters worse, a liver infected with hepatitis C is depleted of glutathione and prone to oxidative damage. A vicious cycle that can lead to cirrhosis has begun.

Liver-biopsy samples from HCV-positive patients have revealed extensive damage resulting from oxidative stress. Milk thistle is a potent free-radical scavenger and has been found to increase the production of glutathione in liver cells. It has also been shown in one animal study to raise glutathione levels by 50 percent.

The value of milk thistle as a free-radical scavenger is not limited to the liver. Although the liver is the main reservoir of glutathione for the whole body, depleted glutathione stores can weaken antioxidant defense systems throughout the body, making us prone to various diseases including cancer.

Milk Thistle Helps to Make New Liver Cells

It's no wonder that milk thistle has remained popular as a liver protector for more than 2,000 years. It blocks the entrance of toxins into the cell and acts as a potent free-radical scavenger. What more can you ask?

Believe it or not, studies have shown that milk thistle promotes the regeneration of hepatocytes. We have previously discussed the amazing regenerating ability of the liver. Milk thistle has actually been shown to support the synthesis of new liver cells that will replace dead and dysfunctional cells.

Arguably, none of the drugs used to treat hepatitis are as valuable as milk thistle at protecting the liver. Its mechanisms of action make a strong case for using milk thistle for hepatitis C. However, many skeptics will still doubt the worth of a substance if it hasn't been tested in humans.

Human Trials Using Milk Thistle to Treat Hepatitis

Silymarin
The therapeutically active compound of milk thistle.

A German study has demonstrated the liver-protecting or antiviral action of milk thistle in hepatitis patients. The study treated 1,000 patients with hepatitis from various causes, including hepatitis B and C, with 140 mg silymarin, the active component in milk thistle, three times daily for three months. The findings included a significant drop in the blood markers for fibrosis, which indicates a lesser amount of disease progression.

Several European trials have shown that milk-thistle extract is beneficial in the management of chronic viral hepatitis. Studies using 420 mg silymarin daily for up to nine months demonstrate a significant decrease in liver enzymes. Liver-biopsy samples taken also show less evidence of liver damage.

The majority of human trials to date have used milk-thistle extracts to treat alcohol-related liver disease and cirrhosis. Several randomized, placebo-controlled trials have confirmed that milk thistle decreases liver enzymes and promotes liver-cell regeneration. A study published in the *Journal of Hepatology* found that 420 mg of silymarin daily improved the four-year survival rate of hepatitis patients with cirrhosis. Moreover, no side effects of silymarin treatment were observed.

How Much Milk Thistle Should You Take?

Milk thistle is a potent liver protector that is virtually devoid of any side effects. It is one of the few herbs that are not contraindicated for pregnant or lactating women. The standard dose of milk thistle is 140 mg three times a day. Clinical improvements are usually noted within eight weeks of starting to take milk thistle. In individuals with chronic liver disease due to hepatitis, ongoing use of milk thistle may be necessary.

Licorice (*Glycyrrhiza glabra*)

In Japan, licorice has been used for more than sixty years as a treatment for hepatitis. Scientists have identified biological activity in more than 50 percent of the licorice plant. *Glycyrrhizin* has been identified as one of the compounds responsible for the anti–hepatitis C activity of licorice.

Stronger Neo-Minophagen, an intravenous (IV) pharmaceutical preparation of *glycyrrhizin*, has been developed to treat hepatitis and other tenacious viruses. Studies have shown that Stronger Neo-Minophagen can profoundly reduce liver inflammation and the damage of hepatitis.

A study published in *The European Journal of Gastroenterology and Hepatology* showed that Stronger Neo-Minophagen significantly lowered liver enzymes, while simultaneously ameliorating cellular evidence of inflammation and necrosis.

Necrosis

Tissue death that occurs in groups of cells in response to a disease process or injury.

Licorice has also been shown to prevent secondary complications of hepatitis, cold sores, and even liver cancer. Licorice's strong antiviral activity provides protection against the viruses that cause the secondary infections resulting from the weakened immune systems found in hepatitis patients. Licorice exhibits antiviral action against the herpes-simplex virus (HSV), human immunodeficiency virus (HIV), *varicella zoster*, and cytomegalovirus (CMV).

How Much Licorice Should You Take?

One thing to be aware of is that licorice supplementation can cause an elevation in blood pressure. This only happens in some people, and the severity depends on the individual, the amount taken, and for how long it is taken. All the symptoms usually disappear when the licorice is stopped.

The benefits of taking licorice for hepatitis outweigh the potential risk of developing elevated blood pressure. When using licorice as an herbal therapy, it's important to monitor your blood pressure regularly, and if it begins to rise, discontinue the licorice treatment.

Individual responses to licorice are highly varied. Finding the appropriate dose is difficult. Nevertheless, 1–5 grams of licorice (containing 2 percent *glycyrrhizin*) daily is a ballpark figure.

Turmeric (*Curcuma longa*)

Dried *Curcuma longa* is the source for the spice

turmeric. Turmeric has been used extensively by Chinese and Ayurvedic doctors for its hepato-protective and anti-inflammatory properties.

The Doctrine of Signatures was an early technique used to explore what herbs to try for different diseases. Herbalists identified the characteristics of plants that correlated with the symptoms of a disease. The characteristic yellow color of dried *Curcuma longa*, as interpreted from the Doctrine of Signatures, was an indication to use it for the yellowing of skin and eyes seen with jaundice.

Herbalists from both India and China, independent of one another, discovered how beneficial turmeric is to the liver. Current research has expanded our understanding of turmeric beyond the Doctrine of Signatures.

The flavonoid curcumin is an active constituent of turmeric. Curcumin has been shown to exhibit antioxidant, anti-inflammatory, anticarcinogenic, and antimicrobial properties. The hepatoprotective effect of turmeric is mainly the result of its antioxidant properties.

Turmeric has been shown to protect the liver from a variety of different toxins, including acetaminophen (Tylenol), carbon tetrachloride, and *Aspergillus aflatoxin* in animals. In one impressive animal study published in *Cancer Letters,* curcumin actually reversed the fatty changes and necrosis induced by *Aspergillus aflatoxin* production.

Alterative Herbs

Milk thistle, licorice, and turmeric are the three herbal medicines most researched for use in hepatitis. They have passed the scientific litmus test with regard to safety and effectiveness. It is incredibly important that herbal medicines be evaluated by modern research; however, we must keep an open mind to other herbs traditionally used to improve liver health.

"Alteratives" are a variety of herbs and can be used to treat liver conditions and enhance liver function. Alteratives are "tonic" herbs that act through various mechanisms to restore a normal balance to the system. They usually act as tonics for the organs of elimination, such as the liver and gallbladder, which, in turn, purify the blood and the lymph.

Three alteratives with a long history of use for sluggish liver and detoxification are dandelion (*Taraxacum officinale*), nettle (*Urtica dioica*), and burdock (*Arctium lappa*). Alteratives nourish and balance the organs of elimination slowly and are usually taken for long periods of time. They are mild and nontoxic and can be considered a healthful part of dietary consumption. Dandelion, nettle, and burdock can be taken as tea or in capsule form. You might also occasionally find dandelion greens and burdock root in the vegetable section of the grocery store.

These alterative herbs are not well-researched for use with hepatitis C. However, their known actions and nontoxic natures make them good candidates for therapy. These herbs have yet to pass the scientific litmus test, but they could some day soon.

CHAPTER 7

BRINGING IT ALL TOGETHER

Are you overwhelmed yet? It's not easy to know where to start. This chapter summarizes the diet, lifestyle, and nutritional and herbal therapies that can help to manage hepatitis.

Herbs

The top three herbal medicines for hepatitis C include milk thistle, licorice, and turmeric. Many other herbs are used to protect the liver and improve its function. However, these three have been shown to be safe and effective in individuals who are positive for HCV.

TABLE 8.1. RECOMMENDED DOSAGES FOR HERBAL MEDICINE	
Herb	**Daily Dosage**
Milk thistle	120–240 mg of standardized extract
Licorice*	$\frac{1}{4}$–$\frac{1}{2}$ teaspoon of licorice-solid extract
Turmeric) (powdered)	1,000 mg three times daily

*Caution: Licorice may raise blood pressure in some individuals.

Vitamins, Minerals, and Other Nutritional Supplements

A high-quality multivitamin serves as nutritional insurance for individuals who are HCV positive. It will prevent nutritional deficiencies that can result in secondary complications of the disease. There are several things to look for when choosing the correct multivitamin, including:

- Avoid iron, unless an iron deficiency is verified by blood work.

- Avoid excess vitamin A; total vitamin A should be between 12,500–25,000 international units (IU), with approximately 2,500 IU of straight vitamin A and the rest from beta-carotene.

- Avoid excess vitamin D; dietary and supplemental vitamin D should not exceed 2,000 IU daily.

- High-quality and high-potency multivitamins should be taken two to three times daily in divided doses.

- Choose brands that are limited to vitamins and minerals; avoid too many added herbs and other ingredients.

- Vitamin E is important enough that it requires special attention. Check the amount of vitamin E in the multivitamin you choose; it is usually 400 IU. If necessary, take additional vitamin E to reach the recommended dose.

A handful of other nutritional supplements should be added to your treatment regime. These include functional foods and other detoxification nutrients. It is important to shop around for good quality; don't settle for substitutions.

TABLE 8.2. RECOMMENDED DOSAGES FOR SUPPLEMENTS	
Supplement	**Daily Dosage**
Vitamin E (d-alpha-tocopherol)	400–800 IU
Whey protein	5 grams
N-acetyl cysteine	500–1,500 mg
Cod-liver oil	2 teaspoons
Alpha-lipoic acid	200–600 mg
Phosphatidyl choline	1,500–2,000 mg

Diet and Lifestyle

Diet provides the foundation for good management of hepatitis C. The following diet guidelines provide a framework for developing your own personalized diet plan.

Eat approximately 2,000–2,500 calories daily consisting of the following:

- Five or more servings of vegetables and fruit.

- Four servings of starchy plants, such as squash, beans, and whole grains.

- Three servings of protein including nuts, seeds, fish, eggs, poultry, lamb, beef, wild game, or pork.

- Two servings of milk, cheese, and yogurt, if tolerated.

- *Avoid caffeine, soda, alcohol, fried and fatty foods, oxidized and synthetic fatty acids, synthetic sweeteners and sugar, additives, preservatives, and coloring agents,*

To maximize liver health, incorporate the following lifestyle advice and rituals into your daily routine:

- Drink plenty of pure water—the number of ounces consumed daily should be half the number of pounds of your body weight. For example, if you weigh 180 pounds, drink 90 ounces of pure water.

- Perform dry-skin brushing (see Chapter 4).

- Apply castor-oil packs two to three times per week (see Chapter 4).

- Exercise thirty to sixty minutes three to four times a week.

- Do breathing exercises (see Chapter 4).

CONCLUSION

Hepatitis C is a chronic liver disease threatening the health of millions of people worldwide. Currently, there are no safe and effective medical treatments available for hepatitis C patients. Drugs used to treat the disease carry serious side effects and have unsatisfactory results.

Conventional medical management for hepatitis C reserves drug treatment until the body shows signs of aggressive liver damage from the hepatitis C virus (HCV). This is because of the potentially serious side effects that can result from the available drug treatments. To make matters worse, drug treatments for hepatitis C are expensive and not covered by many insurance plans.

Hepatitis C can be serious and debilitating. When treatments are ineffective, the disease can lead to cirrhosis and liver failure. HCV reproduces slowly and takes many years before causing disease symptoms. There is a huge window of opportunity within which to start combating HCV by strengthening the body's natural defense against the virus. This is long before HCV causes symptoms of the disease.

The *User's Guide to Treating Hepatitis Naturally* is an educational tool that can increase understanding of HCV and how it affects the body. Understanding the virus, how it is transmitted and how it damages the body, is the first step in successful management of the disease. Know thy enemy! Knowing the characteristics of the HCV also helps to prevent it from spreading.

This book has also introduced you to valuable

herbal, nutritional, dietary, and lifestyle practices that are effective countermeasures to hepatitis C. Herbs such as milk thistle, licorice, and turmeric have passed the scientific litmus test, and one day may be considered part of the standard treatment for hepatitis C. But why wait?

Several nutritional compounds, such as alpha-lipoic acid, vitamin E, whey protein, fish oils, and N-acetyl cysteine, serve as nutritional cofactors that support the liver and immune-system function. In addition, simple diet and lifestyle practices can significantly reduce the work required of the liver and immune system, allowing them to focus on the task at hand—eradicating HCV from the body.

Hepatitis C is not unlike other chronic diseases that slowly erode health and reduce the quality of life. Diet, lifestyle, and environmental factors contribute to the progression and outcome of chronic-disease processes. A proactive approach that focuses on optimal health and nutrition can halt and even reverse the disease process and allow for a good quality of life.

The potentially serious nature of hepatitis C makes it best not to tackle it alone. Seek the help of a qualified team of healthcare practitioners who understand hepatitis C. Combining conventional and alternative approaches will serve you best.

Lab tests and biopsies may be necessary to monitor the disease's progress. However, the doctor you choose should still see you as an individual and not just a combination of diagnostic and lab values. Choose doctors that are open to alternatives and can guide you wisely. The Resources section provides a list of organizations of licensed healthcare practitioners who apply holistic approaches to medicine, as well as some Internet sources of information.

Resources

GreatLife Magazine
Consumer magazine with articles on vitamins, minerals, herbs, and foods.

Available for free at many health and natural food stores.

Let's Live Magazine
Consumer magazine with emphasis on the health benefits of vitamins, minerals, and herbs.

Customer service:
1-800-676-4333
P.O. Box 74908
Los Angeles, CA 90004

Subscriptions: 12 issues per year, $19.95 in the U.S.; $31.95 outside the U.S.

Physical Magazine
Magazine oriented to body builders and other serious athletes.

Customer service:
1-800-676-4333
P.O. Box 74908
Los Angeles, CA 90004

Subscriptions: 12 issues per year, $19.95 in the U.S.; $31.95 outside the U.S.

The Nutrition Reporter™ newsletter
Monthly newsletter that summarizes recent medical research on vitamins, minerals, and herbs.

Customer service:
P.O. Box 30246
Tucson, AZ 85751-0246

e-mail: jack@thenutritionreporter.com
www.nutritionreporter.com

*Subscriptions: $26 per year (12 issues) in the U.S.; $32
U.S. or $48 CNC for Canada; $38 for other countries*

HepNet—The Hepatitis Information Group
www.hepnet.com
*Current information on viral hepatitis A through G
with links to alternative-medicine information.*

Centers for Disease Control (CDC)—Viral Hepatitis Home Page
www.cdc.gov/ncidod/diseases/hepatitis/
*Public information site from the National Center
for Infectious Diseases.*

American Liver Foundation
75 Maiden Lane, Suite 603
New York, NY 10038
Toll free: 800-GO-Liver (465-4837),
888-4HEP-USA (443-7872)
Local: 212-668-1000
Fax: 212-483-8179
www.liverfoundation.org/
*National nonprofit organization promoting liver
health and disease prevention, Provides research,
education, and advocacy for those affected by
hepatitis.*

The American Association of Naturopathic Physicians (AANP)
3201 New Mexico Avenue NW, Suite 350
Washington, DC 20016
Toll free: 866-538-2267
Local: 202-895-1392
Fax: 202-274-1992
www.naturopathic.org
*National professional society representing naturo-
pathic physicians who are licensed or eligible for
licensing as primary-care providers.*

The Institute of Functional Medicine (IFM)
4411 Pt. Fosdick Drive NW, Suite 305
P.O. Box 1697
Gig Harbor, WA 98335
Toll free: 800-228-0622
Fax: 253-853-6766
www.functionalmedicine.org
Organization of healthcare practitioners from several disciplines with a focus on prevention, early assessment, and comprehensive management of complex chronic disease.

American Association of Oriental Medicine (AAOM)
P.O. Box 162340
Sacramento, CA 95816
Toll free: 866-455-7999
Local: 916-443-4770
Fax: 916-443-4766
www.aaom.org
Group of acupuncturists who are committed to high ethical and educational standards and a well-regulated profession to ensure the safety of the public.

American Chiropractic Association
1701 Clarendon Blvd.
Arlington, VA 22209
Toll free: 800-986-4636
Fax: 703-243-2593
www.amerchiro.org/
Group of chiropractors dedicated to providing leadership in health care and a positive vision for the chiropractic profession and its natural approach to health and wellness.

SELECTED
REFERENCES

Arase, Y., K. Ikeda, and N. Murashima. "The long term efficacy of glycyrrhizin in chronic hepatitis C patients." *Cancer,* Vol. 79. (Apr 15 1997): 1494–1500.

Asha, V.V., S. Akhila, P.J. Wills, et al. "Further studies on the antihepatotoxic activity of Phyllanthus maderaspatensis Linn." *Journal of Ethnopharmacology,* Vol. 92. (May 2004): 67–70.

Berkson, B.M. "A Conservative triple antioxidant approach to the treatment of hepatitis C. Combination of alpha-lipoic acid (thiocitic acid), silymarin, and selenium: Three case histories." *Med Klin* (Munich), Vol. 94. (1999): 84–89.

Buzzelli, G., S. Moscarella, A. Giusti, et al. "A pilot study on the liver protective effects of silybin-phosphatidylcholine complex (IdB1016) in chronic active hepatitis." *International Journal of Clinical Pharmacology and Therapeutic Toxicology,* Vol. 31. (Sep 1993): 456–460.

Corrao, G., P.A. Ferrari, and G. Galatola. "Exploring the role of diet in modifying the effect of known disease determinants: application to risk factors of liver cirrhosis." *American Journal of Epidemiology,* Vol. 142. (Dec 1 1995): 1136–1146.

Giese, L.A. "A study of alternative health care use for gastrointestinal disorders." *Gastroenterology Nursing,* Vol. 23. (Jan-Feb 2000): 19–27.

Iino, S., T. Tango, T. Matsushima, et al. "Therapeutic effects of stronger neo-minophagen at different doses on chronic hepatitis and liver cirrhosis." *Hepatology Research,* Vol. 19. (Jan 1 2001): 31–40.

Iwasa, M., K. Iwata, M. Kaito, et al. "Efficacy of long-term dietary restriction of total calories, fat, iron, and protein in patients with chronic hepatitis C virus." *Nutrition*, Vol. 20. (Apr 2004): 368–371.

Leu, G.Z., T.Y. Lin, and J.T. Hsu. "Anti-HCV activities of selective polyunsaturated fatty acids." *Biochemical and Biophysical Research Communications*, Vol. 318. (May 21 2004): 275–280.

Liang, T.J., B. Reherman, L.B. Seef, et al. "Pathogenesis, natural history, treatment and prevention of hepatitis C." *Annals of Internal Medicine*, Vol. 132. (Feb 15 2000): 296–305.

Lieber, C.S., M.A. Leo, K.M. Mak, et al. "Model of non-alcoholic steatohepatitis." *American Journal of Clinical Nutrition*, Vol. 79. (Mar 2004): 502–509.

Lieber, C.S., S.J. Robins, J. Li, et al. "Phosphatidyl-choline protects against fibrosis and cirrhosis in the baboon." *Gastroenterology*, Vol. 106. (Jan 1994): 152–159.

Milliman, W.B., D.W. Lamson, and M.S. Brignall. "Hepatitis C: a retrospective study, literature review, and naturopathic protocol." *Alternative Medicine Review*, Vol. 5. (Aug 2000): 355–371.

Moscarella, S., A. Giusti, F. Marra, et al. "Therapeutic and antilipoperoxidant effects of silybin-phosphatidyl-choline complex in chronic liver disease: preliminary results." *Current Therapeutic Research*, Vol. 53. (1993): 98–102.

Niederau, C., G. Strohmeyer, T. Heintges, et al. "Polyunsaturated phosphatidyl-choline and interferon alpha for treatment of chronic hepatitis B and C: a multi-center, randomized, double-blind, placebo-controlled trial." Leich study group. *Hepatogastroenterology*, Vol. 45. (May-Jun 1998): 797–804.

Okada, S., K. Tanaka, T. Sato, et al. "Dose-response trial of lactoferrin in patients with chronic hepatitis C." *Japanese Journal of Cancer Research*, Vol. 93. (Sep 2002): 1063–1069.

Patrick, L. "Hepatitis C: epidemiology and review of complementary/alternative medicine treatments." *Alternative Medicine Review*, Vol. 4. (Aug 1999): 220–238.

Salmon, S. "Herbs and Hepatitis C." *International Journal of Complementary and Alternative Medicine,* (Sept 1997): 24–26.

Sarbah, S.A., and Z.M. Younossi. "Hepatitis C: An update on the silent epidemic." *Journal of Clinical Gastroenterology,* Vol. 30. (Mar 2000): 125–143.

Suarez, M., O. Beloqui, J.V. Fererr, et al. "Glutathione depletion in chronic hepatitis C." *Intl Hepatol Commun,* Vol. 1. (1993): 215–221.

Teo, M., and P. Hayes. "Management of hepatitis C." *British Medical Bulletin,* Vol. 70. (Oct 2004): 51–69.

Watanabe, A., K. Okada, Y. Shimizu, et al. "Nutritional therapy of chronic hepatitis C by whey protein (non-heated)." *Journal of Medicine,* Vol. 31. (2000): 283–302.

INDEX

Printed in the USA
CPSIA information can be obtained
at www.ICGtesting.com
JSHW051957150824
68134JS00050B/91